Nutrition for Healing the Body in Recovery Unlocked:

Nutritional guide for Healing and Recovering your body

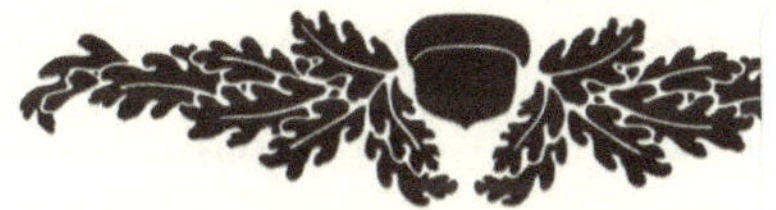 

BY Z.D Snee

It is creative nonfiction, in this case. For various reasons, several parts have undergone variable degrees of fictionalization.

TABLE OF CONTENTS

<u>DISCLAIMER</u>

Are you feeling lost and stressed out as you try to heal? This isn't just another cookbook; it's your warm hug and personalized plan to get you back on track. We can help you do well by giving you tasty food, strong tactics, and a friendly community. Inside, you'll find a collection of tasty, easy-to-follow recipes that are meant to feed your body and help you heal. You can find healthy and filling choices for every meal, from breakfasts that will wake you up to dinners that will make you feel good. They are all full of the nutrients you need to feel your best. But food isn't just power. It's an exciting world of food synergy where-putting certain items together can reveal health benefits you didn't know about. Discover useful foods that are made to help with certain issues and look into how personalized nutrition can give you the power to take charge of your health and well-being. Healing is a process, not a place you get to. This book has more than just ideas. We'll give you the tools you need to feel comfortable in social situations, deal with stress well, and get enough sleep first. These are all basic things you should do to heal fully. Are you feeling too much? We'll show you how to make friends who will help you and how to celebrate your wins, no matter how big or small they are. You can build a bright and healthy future one tasty meal and empowering plan at a time if you are kind to yourself and think positively. Are you ready to start your healing journey with a group of people who will help you? Let's do it together!

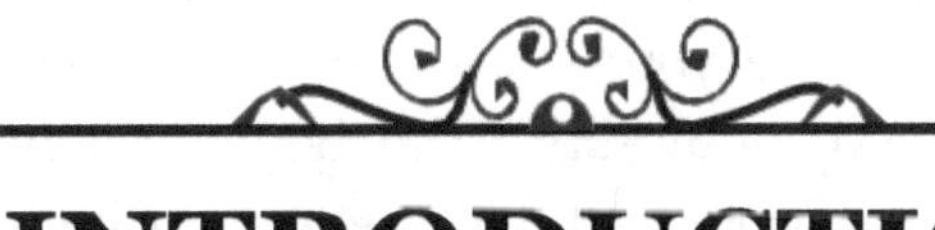
INTRODUCTION

Ignite Your Inner Healer

"Incredible power of food to unlock your body's natural healing potential."

Do you ever really want to heal, to get back the healthy energy and happiness that you may have been missing for a while? Now, fasten your seat belts causing you to have the key to unlocking the amazing power of food! Your body's natural ability to heal itself is hidden in the colorful world of fruits, veggies, whole grains, and lean proteins, just waiting to be released. Think of your body as a beautiful machine that can fix itself. It's always working to restore damaged cells, protect itself from outside threats, and build itself back up stronger. But food is what makes this amazing process possible. You can take an active role in your own healing by picking the right foods. These foods will bring out your inner healer and give your body the tools it needs to thrive. Picture a cut or scrape on your skin. Your body already has the tools you need to heal it. However, wouldn't it help your body heal faster if you gave it the building blocks it needs? The same idea applies to healing from the inside out. By eating foods that are high in zinc, vitamin C, and protein, you give your body the building blocks it needs to heal itself quickly. But food has more power than just giving us building blocks. Think of your gut as a busy environment full of trillions of tiny microbes, some good and some bad. These bacteria are very important for digestion, the immune system, and even controlling mood. By feeding good bacteria foods like whole grains, fruits, and veggies that are high in prebiotics, you create a healthy gut environment that helps your body heal and stay healthy. This diet isn't hard to follow or complex. It means opening up to a world of colorful, tasty foods that are good for your body and mind. Think of it as a journey through food, where each bite is a step towards being your best self. Think of sweet berries that are full of antioxidants, leafy greens that are full of vitamins, and lean meats that help build strong muscles. Instead of just being a source of calories, it's about praising food as a powerful way to heal.

You might not have to go in a straight line to find your inner healer. Things will go wrong sometimes, and days will come when your needs win. Life will also throw you some curve balls you didn't see coming. However, the most important thing is to be kind and patient with yourself during the process. Every meal that is good for you is a step in the right direction. Your body can fix itself in amazing ways, and when you work with the power of food, you can unlock its full potential and start a life-changing journey towards vibrant health and well-being. Are you ready to bring out your inner therapist and take back your healing power? Let the tasty adventure begin!

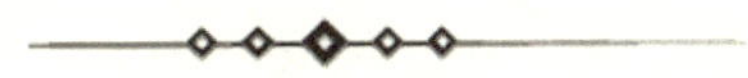

Embrace the Journey

*"Get ready for a transformative adventure
towards a healthier, happier you."*

Ever wished for a life full of energy, where your body felt like a well-oiled machine, and your heart soared with newfound life? Maybe your goal is to get rid of tiredness and aches and to finally feel completely at ease in your own skin. This, my friend, isn't just a dream; it's an adventure waiting to happen. The key is to be open to the life-changing trip that will make you healthier and happier. It's kind of like starting a big adventure. This epic adventure needs a plan, a desire to explore, and a readiness to accept the unexpected, just like any other epic adventure. Each person's plan is unique, with a mix of diet, exercise, and self-care that works for them. Your curiosity about new healthy habits and your eagerness to find out what amazing things your body can do will fuel your trip. And those sudden turns? They will happen, but if you have the right attitude, you can turn them into chances to learn and grow. The path ahead might not be a sprint to the finish line. It's a lovely, winding road where you can find lots of interesting things. You might see a secret gem, like a healthy and tasty recipe that everyone in the family loves. You might find out you have a strength you didn't know you had, like the ability to do a hard yoga pose or say no to sweets. It's these wins, no matter how big or small, that make the journey so worthwhile. The great thing is that you're not on this journey by yourself. There are a lot of people out there who share your passion for good living. You can join online communities, take exercise classes, or look for a friend who shares your goals and can help you reach them. This sense of community keeps you going and makes you realize that you're a part of something bigger than yourself. You might need to make small changes over time to become healthy. You could switch from sugary drinks to fruit-flavored sparkling water or from processed snacks to a handful of almonds. Every change, no matter how small it seems, is a step in the right way. Always being the same is important. A daily walk, even if it's only for 15 minutes, is better for you than doing hard workouts once in a while. Keep your eyes on the big wins because the little ones lead to the bigger ones.

Allow yourself to be surprised by how you change as you go along the trip. You might fall in love with cooking all over again, find joy in mindful movement, or realize how strong your body really is. You don't just want to get to the end of this trip; you want to enjoy the process of becoming healthier and happier. So, pack your bags with excitement, a little wonder, and a lot of kindness for yourself. There's an exciting journey ahead of you that will lead to a better you.

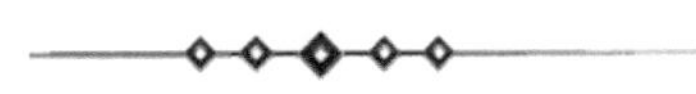

Let Food Be Your Medicine

"Learn how to harness the power of nutrition to support your body's recovery journey."

You feel a little under the weather and slow. You may even be dealing with a health issue. When you go to the doctor, you hope to find a magic pill that will take away all of your problems. Why take a pill if the answer is your food, which you know better? Some people may think this is too good to be true, but food can be some of the best medicine possible. By using nutrition to its fullest, you can help your body heal itself and get back to being healthy and happy. Imagine that your body is a wonderful machine that can fix itself. It's always working in the background to repair damaged cells, protect itself from outside threats, and grow stronger. But, like any machine, it needs the right fuel to work at its best. This is where food comes in. By picking the right foods, you give your body the building blocks and nutrients it needs to heal quickly.

Let's use protein as an example. Every cell in your body is built on top of it, and it's very important for healing tissues and making your immune system healthy. Adding protein-rich foods to your diet, like lean meats, fish, eggs, and beans, is a proactive way to help your body heal. It's not just protein, though. There are a lot of vitamins, minerals, and antioxidants in a rainbow of fruits and veggies. As your body's internal cheerleaders, these strong micronutrients boost its defenses and fight inflammation. They're like little soldiers whose job it is to keep you safe. And the gut! This secret ecosystem is full of trillions of microbes that help with digestion, immunity, and even mood. When you eat foods like whole grains, fruits, and veggies that are high in prebiotics, you feed the good bacteria in your gut and make it a healthy place that helps your body heal.

Using food as healing is great because it looks at the whole person. You're not just healing one symptom; you're giving your body what it needs to heal itself from the inside out. Being proactive about your health and taking an active role in your healing is the best way to do it.

This trip might not always go as planned. Some days, your hunger will win, or life will throw you a curveball you didn't see coming. However, the most important thing is to be kind and patient with yourself during the process. Every meal that is good for you is a step in the right direction.

Food is more than just fuel; it's a way to celebrate. Enjoy the bright colors on your plate, the tasty flavors that tempt your taste buds, and the amazing power of food to heal and feed your body. Come up with new recipes and enjoy making healthy meals. Let your home become a healing and well-being haven. Don't let medicine hurt you; let food heal you, and start getting healthier and happier!

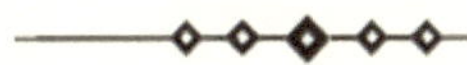

CHAPTER 1

The Healing Powerhouse

"Macronutrients"

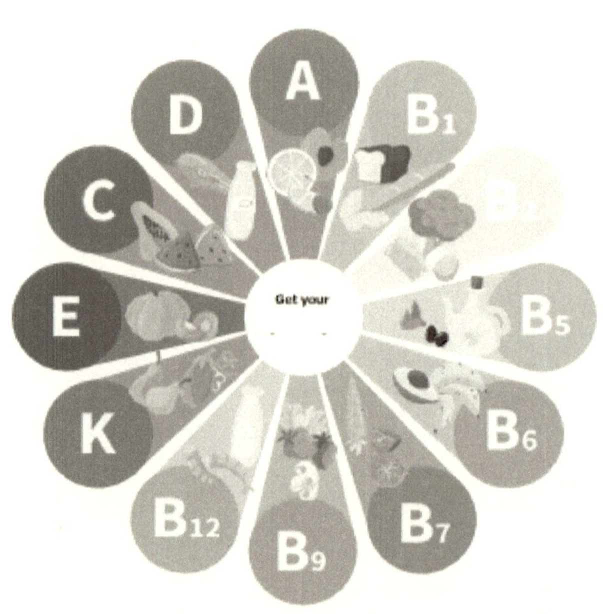

Fueling Your Recovery

"Explore the essential macronutrients (carbs, protein, fat) and their role in rebuilding your body."

Think of your body as a beautiful building place. Like a group of hardworking builders, it's always trying to fix, rebuild, and get stronger. But for this crew to do its job well, it needs the right tools. Step into the world of macronutrients, which are carbs, protein, and fat. These are the building blocks that your body needs to heal itself.

Carbs are what give you energy.

Let's picture carbs as your body's main source of power. Your body needs carbs to power its daily processes, just like construction workers need a steady supply of energy to keep going. When you eat these carbs, your body breaks them down into glucose, which gives your cells, muscles, and brain energy quickly. Complex carbs are found in large amounts in whole grains, fruits, and veggies. They slowly provide you with power over time, which keeps you going all day.

The building blocks of life are proteins.

Think about those builders who needed bricks to build the walls. Yes, that's what protein does! A protein is made up of amino acids, which are the building blocks of hormones, enzymes, and cells in your body. Your body needs the right amount of protein to heal damaged cells, build new muscle, and keep your immune system strong while you're recovering. Foods like lean meats, fish, eggs, beans, and cheese are all great sources of protein that can help your body heal.

Fat: Not the Enemy, But a Valuable Friend

Fat gets a bad name a lot of the time, but it's very important for healing. Eating healthy fats is important for making hormones, absorbing nutrients, and keeping cells healthy. They also give you long-lasting energy and help you feel full after a meal. Healthy fats from foods like nuts, seeds, avocado, and olive oil are like cement that holds the building blocks (protein) together and keeps the structure (your body) strong and healthy.

How to Find the Right Balance

Now, getting these macronutrients isn't enough to help you heal; you also need to find the right balance between them. This balance can change based on your unique needs and where you are in your recovery. But eating whole, unprocessed things is a good place to start. Put colorful fruits and veggies on your plate, along with lean protein sources and healthy fats in small amounts. Why these macronutrients don't work alone is because of "the power of synergy." They work together in a way that makes them more effective. For instance, mixing protein with carbs can help build and fix muscles. Adding healthy fats to food makes it even easier for the body to absorb nutrients. To give your body everything it needs to heal and grow, you need to make sure that these macro-nutrients are balanced.

This way of fueling your healing isn't about dieting or counting calories very carefully. Getting aware and taking charge of your healing journey is what it's all about. When you know what macronutrients do and choose healthy foods, you give your body the tools it needs to heal, rebuild, and come back stronger than ever. Learn about healthy foods, try out new meals that look good, and fuel your recovery the right way: by eating a balanced diet of macronutrients!

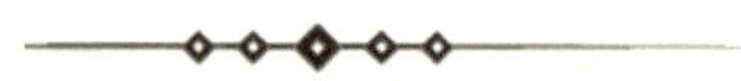

Building Blocks of Strength

"Understand how protein supports tissue repair and strengthens your immune system."

Think of your body as a beautiful fortress that is always working to stay strong and protect itself from outside threats. But what if the walls of this fortress were broken because someone was sick or hurt? Protein is like a superhero because it helps fix damaged tissues and boosts your immune system, which are two important parts of a strong and healthy body. Protein is like the building blocks of life. It's a very important part of building and repairing muscles, enzymes, hormones, and tissues. Protein is important for the structure and operation of every cell in your body. For example, your body needs a lot more protein when it's recovering from an accident, surgery, or even just a lot of hard training. Let's look at how protein can help you heal in more detail:

The Tissue Repair Crew

Picture a building crew working hard to fix cracks in a wall. Proteins are also the building blocks that your body uses to restore damaged tissues. Protein is used by your body to rebuild muscle fibers, heal wounds, and grow new skin over broken skin. Making sure that this repair crew eats enough protein gives them the tools they need to do the job quickly.

Powerhouse of Muscle

The muscles that power you through the day are like engines. Protein is very important for building and repairing muscles while you're recovering, especially after an injury that hurts your muscles. Proteins are made up of amino acids, which are used to rebuild and strengthen muscle cells. This makes them stronger and better able to do their job.

Ally for the Immune System

Your immune system is like an army that fights off bacteria and viruses that try to get into your body. Protein is necessary to make antibodies, which are the immune system's fighters that find and kill these invaders. By making sure you get enough protein, you give your body the tools it needs to fight off illness

and infection.

The Freedom to Choose

The next question is where to find this special protein. Nature, on the other hand, has a lot of tasty protein-rich foods that can help you get better. Eggs and dairy products, as well as lean meats like chicken, fish, and turkey, are all great picks. Nuts, tofu, lentils, beans, and other legumes are great plant-based sources of protein.

More Than the Basics

Getting enough protein is important, but it's also important to pay attention to the quality of the protein sources you eat. Most of the time, your body can absorb and use lean, raw foods better than processed meats or fried foods. To make sure you get all the amino acids you need, you might also want to eat different kinds of protein throughout the day. Building a body that is strong and durable takes time. When it comes to protein, consistency is very important. Getting protein at different times of the day, like with meals and snacks, makes sure that your body always has this important building block.

Learn about the benefits of protein and plan how to include it in your diet.

This will not only help you recover, but it will also build a body that is healthy and strong. Learn about the world of protein-rich foods, try out some tasty recipes, and give your body the tools it needs to get stronger than ever.

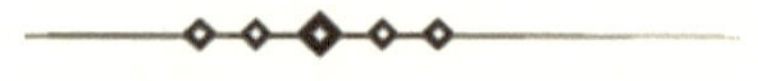

Unleashing Energy

"Learn how carbohydrates provide the fuel your body needs for healing and daily activities."

Think of your body as a car that needs to find its way back to health. It needs the right food to keep going, to do daily tasks, and to help very important healing processes. That's where carbohydrates come in; they are the main fuel that your body's engine runs on. Carbs give you energy to keep going strong, while protein helps you build muscle. You can think of carbs as the easy-to-find food that your body can turn into glucose. Your brain, muscles, and cells get most of their energy from this glucose. It gives you the power to do everyday things, like going up and down stairs or working out hard. It's even more important to eat enough carbs during healing when your body is working hard to fix itself. Here are some ways that carbs can help you heal:

Energy to Fix Things

In the same way that a building site needs electricity to run its tools, your body needs energy to heal itself. When you are sick or hurt, carbohydrates give your body the power it needs to do important things. This frees up your body's re- sources so it can heal cells and fight off infections.

Replenishment of muscle glycogen

During hard workouts or times of physical stress, your muscles use glycogen for energy. Glycogen is a form of glucose that is stored in your muscles and is easy to access. Carbohydrates help muscles rebuild glycogen stores that have been used up during recovery, especially after strenuous exercise. This makes sure that your muscles have the energy they need to work well and heal properly.

Better Mood and Focus

Have you ever had that awful "brain fog" when you haven't eaten enough? That sounds like your brain is sending out an SOS! To work right, your brain needs a a lot of glucose for energy. Eating enough carbohydrates helps keep blood sugar levels in a healthy range, which can improve brain function, focus, and even mood control. This can help a lot during healing when you may be feeling more stressed out and tired.

Be Smart About Your Choices—Not All Carbs Are the Same

There are different kinds of carbs. Simple carbs are quickly broken down and can be found in sugary drinks, white bread, and sweets. They cause blood sugar to rise and then drop. You might feel tired and want more sugar after this. Complex carbs, on the other hand, like those in whole grains, fruits, and veggies, are broken down more slowly but give you energy over a longer period. For your healing, these are the carbs you should eat the most of.

Getting Your Day Going:

So, how do you add these powerful sources of energy to your diet? Throughout the day, try to eat a range of whole, unprocessed carbs. Whole carbs, like brown rice or quinoa, go well with lean protein sources. Every meal, eat a mixed plate of fruits and veggies. These options will give your body a steady flow of energy, which will keep you fed and alert while you heal.

It's not bad for your body to eat carbs. Selecting the correct kinds of carbs and arranging them in a smart way in your diet will not only give you energy for daily tasks, but it will also help your body heal. Let go of the sweets, eat more whole grains and vegetables, and let the power of carbs fuel your trip back to health!

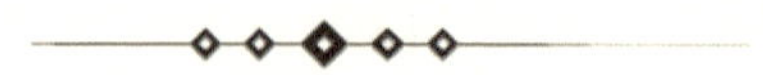

CHAPTER 2

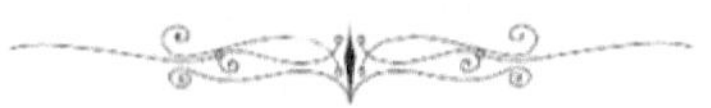

Gut Feeling

"Nourishing Your Mind & Body"

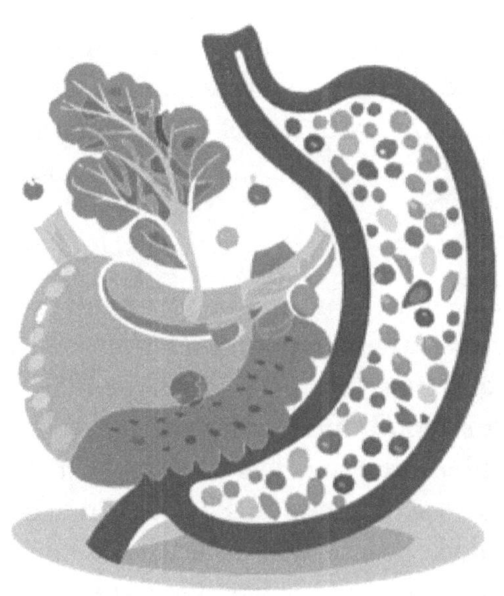

The Gut-Brain Connection Revealed

"The fascinating link between your gut health and mental well-being."

People have been taught for a long time that the gut is only where our food is processed. New science discoveries, on the other hand, have shown an interesting twist: your gut and brain are directly connected and can have a big effect on your mental health. Hold on tight because we're about to dive into the gut-brain axis and look at how a healthy gut can make you happy. Imagine that your gut is a busy city full of trillions of tiny people, both good and bad germs. These bacteria are very important for digestion, getting nutrients into the body, and even immune system health. The amazing thing is that they can also talk to your brain! A complicated web of nerves, hormones, and immune cells makes this contact possible. Neurotransmitters are chemicals that your brain cells use to talk to each other. They are made by the good bacteria in your gut. These hormones can change how you feel, how stressed you are, and even how you sleep. This means that when your gut is happy and healthy, with lots of good bacteria, it can send good messages to your brain that make you feel good and strong.

The Bad Things About Having an Unhappy Gut

Let's do the opposite now. Your brain and gut microbiome can't talk to each other properly if there are too many bad bacteria in your gut. Eventually, this can cause your body to make inflammatory chemicals that can hurt your mood and brain function. You could feel more anxious, have trouble thinking clearly, or even start to show signs of sadness. How can we strengthen this link and make sure our guts are happy, which is good for our mental health? What we eat is the key. That's how prebiotics work; they feed your gut garden. They feed the good bacteria, which helps them grow and pushes out the bad ones. Prebiotics can be found in large amounts in fruits, veggies, and whole grains. Fermented foods, like kimchi, yogurt, and kombucha, are full of live and active cultures, which are good bacteria that help keep your gut microbiome healthy.

Limit processed foods, sugar, and fats that are bad for you. These can throw off the balance in your gut, helping bad bacteria grow and stopping good ones from doing their job. Water is important for gut health because it aids digestion and the uptake of nutrients. Keeping yourself hydrated is good for your gut.

Besides Food

A whole-person method is key, even though diet is very important. Your gut health can get worse if you're stressed all the time. Meditation, yoga, and spending time in nature are all good ways to deal with stress and keep your gut healthy. Not getting enough sleep can hurt your gut microbiome. To keep your gut and brain healthy, try to get 7-8 hours of good sleep every night. While more research needs to be done, some studies show that taking probiotic pills may have extra health benefits for your gut and help keep your mood in check. Before you start taking any vitamins, talk to your doctor.

By taking care of your gut and promoting a healthy gut microbiome, you're not only improving digestion and nutrient absorption, but you're also making your mind happy and stronger. Your gut is an important part of your health and not just a place to process food. So please pay attention to your gut and feed it the right things. Your brain will thank you!

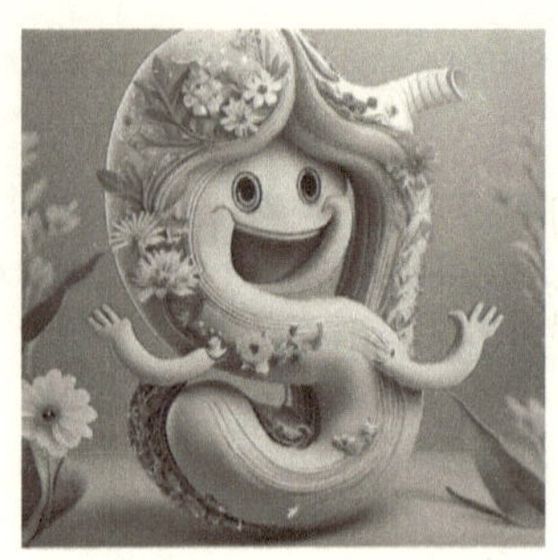

Fueling Your Happy Gut

"What foods nourish your gut microbiome and promote emotion- al balance."

Your gut microbiome is like a lively inner world full of trillions of tiny living things. There are both good and bad bacteria living in your gut. They play an interesting role in both digestion and your general health. A new study shows an interesting link between the health of your gut and how you feel. So, let's talk about how to keep your emotions in check and feed your happy gut with tasty foods. You can think of the microbiome in your gut as a busy environment. The good bacteria take care of the surroundings and keep the bad bacteria in check, like good gardeners. A complex network of nerves and chemicals tells your brain that everything is okay when this happy balance is strong. These cues can make you feel better, help you handle stress better, and even help you sleep better. Your gut bacteria need prebiotics to grow, just like a garden needs rich dirt. These fibers that can't be digested feed the good bacteria, which helps them grow and beat out the bad ones. Luckily, nature is full of prebiotic-rich foods that can keep your gut healthy: Enjoy the colors of the rainbow!

There are a lot of prebiotics in fruits and vegetables. Fruits like berries, apples, and bananas, and veggies like artichokes, asparagus, and leafy greens. Give up white bread and eat whole grains instead, like oats, brown rice, and quinoa. These are full of prebiotic fiber, which makes your gut happy and calms you down. Not only are beans, lentils, and chickpeas high in protein, but they are also high in prebiotics. They can help keep your gut and mind healthy. Foods that have been fermented, like cabbage, kimchi, yogurt, and kombucha, are like probiotics on steroids. These foods are full of live and active cultures, which are good bacteria that help keep your gut microbiome healthy. Not only do they help your gut, but they can also improve your mood and make you feel more emotionally stable. Fiber is essential, so don't forget about it! Fiber not only helps your body digest food and makes you feel full, but it also feeds the good bugs in your gut. Add whole grains to your meals, eat fruits and veggies with the skins still on, and snack on nuts and seeds to get more fiber and keep your gut healthy.

Pay attention to what you leave out.

It's important to eat these gut-friendly foods, but it's also important to avoid things that can throw off the balance in your gut. A lot of processed foods are low in fiber and high in sugar and fats, which are bad for you. These things can hurt the bacteria in your gut and make mood swings and worry worse. Sugar feeds the bad bugs in your gut, which can throw off your balance and maybe even affect how you feel. Watch out for added sugar, and choose fruits and veggies that are naturally sweet. Some fats are necessary for health, but too much of the bad fats found in processed foods and fried foods can be bad for your gut. Pick healthy fats, like those in olive oil, nuts, seeds, bananas, and other nuts and seeds.

Beyond Food: Taking Care of Your Inner Ecosystem

It's not just the food you eat that keeps your gut healthy. Gut bacteria can get messed up by long-term worry. Meditation, yoga, and spending time in nature are all good ways to deal with stress and help your gut bacteria grow. Not get- ting enough sleep can hurt your gut health. To keep your gut and brain healthy, try to get 7-8 hours of good sleep every night. It has been shown that regular exercise is good for your gut bacteria. Do something you enjoy most days of the week, like dancing, swimming, brisk walks, or something else.

By giving your gut the right foods, dealing with stress, and putting a healthy lifestyle first, you're not only improving digestion, but you're also taking steps towards a more stable and strong mental state. Eat tasty foods that are high in prebiotics, learn more about the benefits of fermented foods, and take care of your gut. Your body and mind will thank you.

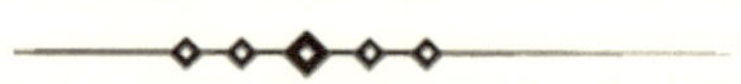

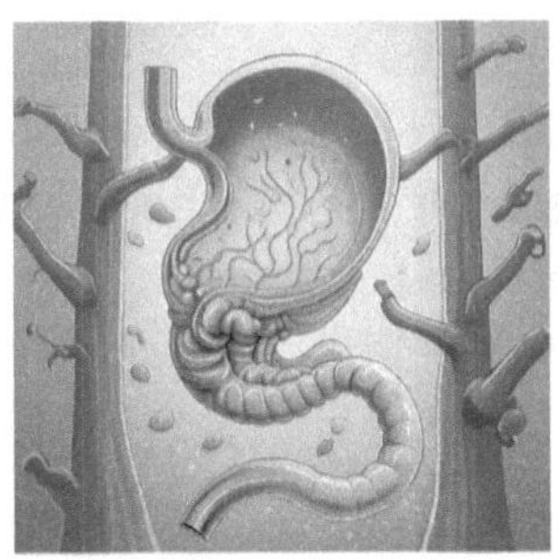

Taming the Tummy Troubles

*"Learn strategies to overcome digestive issues
and support overall gut health."*

Feeling bloated, gassy, or having painful stomach cramps is something that many people experience. If so, you're not the only one! Many people have problems with their digestion, which can make them sick or take away from their pleasure in life. But before you give up and accept a lifetime of pain, there is good news: you can get rid of those stomach problems and support a healthy gut by making changes to your food and lifestyle and doing some research. The gut is a complicated environment full of trillions of bacteria, some good and some bad. Digestive problems can happen when this careful balance is thrown off. Anything from worry and anxiety to food allergies and a bad diet could be to blame. This is where the foods you eat can help calm a stomach that is giving you trouble. Find out if you have food sensitivities. Some foods can make your stomach react badly. You could write down what you eat and how you feel afterwards in a food notebook. This can help you figure out what might be causing your symptoms, like lactose intolerance or gluten sensitivity. In your gut, fiber works like a gentle broom to support digestion and keep your bowel movements normal.

To keep things running easily, eat a lot of fiber-rich fruits, vegetables, and whole grains. Water is very important for digestion. To keep your gut system healthy and working right, try to drink a lot of water throughout the day. Probiotics are live cultures that can help your gut bacteria get back in balance. You could add fermented foods like kimchi, yogurt, and kombucha to your diet, or you could talk to your doctor about probiotic pills. When you eat too much, your gut system can't handle it. Pay attention to your body's hunger signals and stop eating before you feel too full to move.

After the Plate

Food is an important part of the equation, but it's also important to look at the whole picture. Long-term stress can be very bad for your gut health. Spending time in nature, meditating, or doing deep breathing exercises can help you deal with stress and keep your digestive system calm. Not getting enough sleep can hurt the bacteria in your gut. Aim for 7-8 hours of good sleep every night to keep your gut and general health in good shape. Regular exercise can help keep your gut moving and keep you from getting constipated. Do things you enjoy, like walks, swimming, or dancing, and make it a point to move around most days of the week. Don't be afraid to get professional help if your stomach problems don't go away no matter what you do. Talking to a doctor or qualified dietitian can help you figure out what's causing your gut health problems and make a plan just for you.

Getting rid of stomach problems takes time and a willingness to try new things. You can take back control of your gut health and live a life without stomach pain by figuring out what works for you, making smart food choices, and adopting healthy habits. Enjoy the trip, pay attention to your body's messages, and start making changes from the inside out to become happier and healthier.

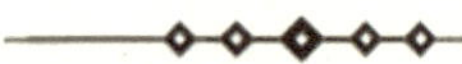

CHAPTER 3

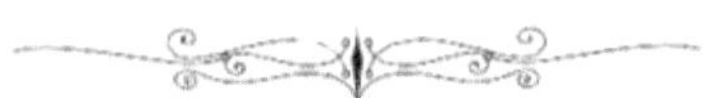

Your Personalized Recipe

"For Recovery"

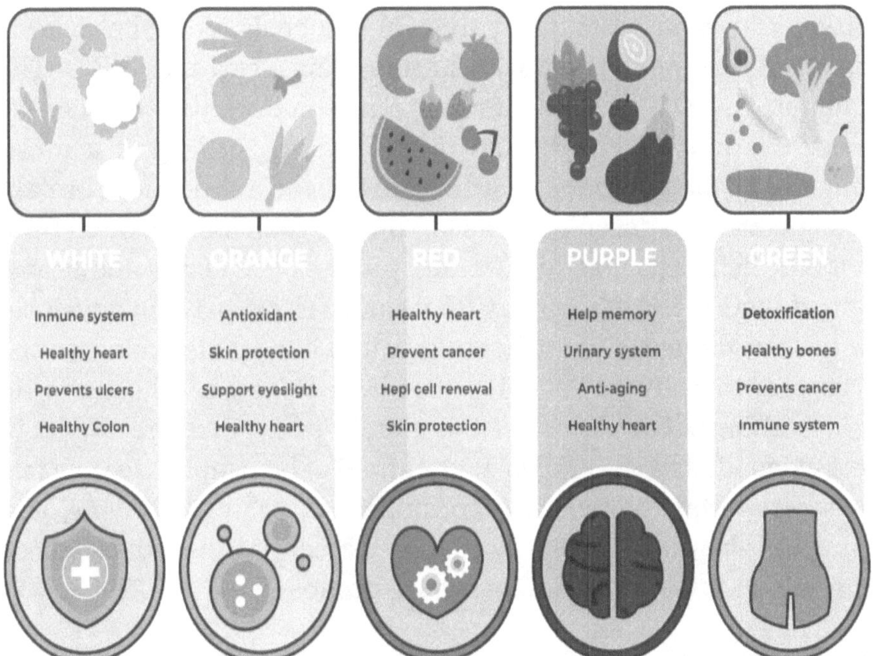

Unlocking Your Body's Needs

"How to tailor your nutrition plan based on your unique recovery goals."

Think of your body as a beautiful machine that is always trying to fix, rebuild, and improve itself. But, like any machine, it needs the right fuel to work at its best. This is where personalized nutrition really shines! By figuring out what your body needs to heal, you can make a nutrition plan that helps you get back to being at your healthiest, whether you're recovering from a disease, injury, surgery, or just training hard. There is no one way to get better. Are you getting better from a certain injury, like an ankle sprain? You might be getting better after surgery. Or maybe you're an athlete who wants to get the most out of your recovery after a run. The first step in making a personalized nutrition plan is to write down your unique goals. Your diet plan is made up of macronutrients, which are proteins, carbs, and fats. The best amount of each of these nutrients relies on what your body needs to heal. For muscle growth and tissue healing, protein is a must. During the healing process, your body may need a little more protein than someone who doesn't do much. You can get a lot of protein from lean foods, fish, eggs, and plant-based proteins like lentils and beans. Your body gets most of its energy from carbs. The kind of sugar you eat does matter, though. Choose complex carbs like whole grains, fruits, and veggies that give you energy that lasts so you can heal and do everyday things. Cut down on the simple carbs that are found in processed foods and sweets. Do not be afraid of fat people! Healthy fats are very important for making hormones, absorbing nutrients, and keeping cells healthy. To help you get better, eat healthy fats like those in olive oil, nuts, seeds, avocados, and avocados.

Beyond the Basics: Micronutrients Are Important Too!

Micronutrients, like vitamins and minerals, are also important for your body to work at its best. Here are some important people for recovery:

Vitamin C: This vitamin powerhouse helps the body heal tissues and keep its immune system healthy. You should eat leafy veggies, citrus fruits, and berries.

Vitamin D: Vitamin D is needed for strong bones and a healthy immune system. You can get it from fatty fish, eggs, and foods that have been enriched, like milk and cereals.

Iron: This element is very important for moving oxygen around the body, which is needed for healing and making energy. Iron can be found in large amounts in beans, leafy greens, and lean foods. Foods that are high in zinc, like red meat, chicken, and seafood, can help wounds heal and keep your immune system strong.

Pay attention to your body.

Your plan is like a road map, but your body gives you important signs. Listen to your body when it tells you it's hungry or full. If you're always tired or slow, you might need to change how many calories you eat. If you have problems with your digestion, you might want to change the kinds of fiber you're eating. Healthy habits and a good diet go hand in hand. Aim for enough sleep, learn how to relax to deal with stress, and drink plenty of water throughout the day. These habits will help you get better even faster. A trained dietitian can help you figure out what to eat. They can help you make a plan that fits your needs and enables you to reach your healing goals, taking into account things like food allergies and preferences.

When you take the time to figure out what your body needs and make a personalized nutrition plan, you're not only fueling your healing; you're also giving yourself the tools you need to take charge of your health. Take a look at personalized nutrition, pay attention to your body, and start your road to a healthier, stronger you!

Bio individuality

"One Size Doesn't Fit All: Learn why finding personalized solutions is key to optimal healing."

When you look through a magazine with "one-size-fits-all" exercise or diet plans, do you ever get a bad feeling? You may have tried them but found that they made you feel tired or unhappy. The truth is that everyone's body is different, so what works great for one person might not be great for someone else. This is where the interesting idea of bio-individuality comes in: the notion that there is no one perfect way to heal or be healthy. Imagine that a group of friends are getting better after getting hurt. It works great for one person, but it makes another person feel sluggish. There's nothing wrong with this; it's just bio-individuality at work. How our bodies handle food and recover from stress is affected by things like our genes, the health of our guts, and how active we are.

Why bio-individuality is important

To heal, different kinds of accidents need other nutrients. For muscle repair, a sprained ankle might need more protein, while a broken bone might do better with calcium and vitamin D. A bio-individual method makes sure that you give your body the exact nutrients it needs to heal quickly. The trillions of bacteria that live in your gut are very important for digestion, getting nutrients into your body, and even your defense system. Your gut bacteria can be changed by what you eat in a big way. If you know how healthy your gut is, you can change your food to support a healthy gut environment, which can help your body heal even more. Of course, some people burn calories faster than others. This means that a "one-size-fits-all" 2000-calorie diet could make some people feel hungry all the time, while it could make others gain weight. Bio-individuality looks at your unique metabolic rate to make sure your body has the energy it needs to heal without cutting calories too much. You are the only one who knows your body best. Bio-individuality tells you to pay attention to what your body is telling you. Are you tired after eating a certain thing? Change what you eat. Have trouble with bloating after eating some vegetables? Try out different options. If you pay attention to what your body is telling you, you can choose foods that will help you heal.

Putting bio-individuality into practice

A doctor or registered dietitian can help you figure out what you need based on your health history, current condition, and level of exercise. They will be able to help you make a plan for your own healing. Food allergies that aren't obvious can sometimes get in the way of healing. You could write down how you feel after eating different foods in a food notebook. By doing this, you can find possible triggers and change your food to avoid them. Supplements may be helpful, but whole, raw foods that give your body the nutrients it needs should be your first choice. Healthy fats, lean proteins, fruits, and veggies make up the main parts of a personalized detox diet. To reach your best health, you need to run a race, not a sprint. It's okay that the road will have bumps. Have a growth attitude, try new things, and pay attention to how your body reacts.

What is the Power of Customized Healing? When you accept bio-individuality, you move away from rigid, one-size-fits-all plans and towards a personalized method that respects your unique body. You can take charge of your health and healing journey when you feel this way. The best way to heal is not to use a one-size-fits-all method but to unlock your body's potential and find the answers that work best for you. So, pay attention to your body, look into personalized choices, and start a healing journey that is made just for you!

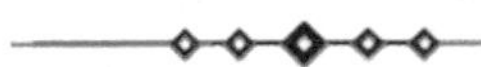

Embarking on Your Culinary Adventure

"Explore various dietary approaches and find the one that resonates with your body and taste buds."

Imagine that your life is a food adventure! Food isn't just fuel; it's a way to try new tastes, learn about other countries, and, most importantly, discover what your body needs. There is no one "right" way to eat when it comes to different methods. The important thing is to go on an adventure of discovery, trying out different choices until you find the one that works best for your body and tastes good.

A World of Delicious Foods

This way of thinking stresses balance and variety. It tells you to eat a variety of fruits and veggies, whole grains for long-lasting energy, lean proteins for repair and growth, and healthy fats to feel full and absorb nutrients. This is an open-ended method that lets you make your food fit your tastes and health goals. This diet is based on the usual ways of eating in countries that are close to the Mediterranean Sea. It emphasizes healthy fats like olive oil, fruits, vegetables, whole grains, and fish. It's known to be good for your heart and general health. This is "The Vegetarian Adventure." This method doesn't use meat and instead focuses on protein-rich plants like nuts, beans, lentils, tofu, and tempeh. Getting more fruits, veggies, and fiber can be easy if you do this. Make sure you get enough protein and important nutrients like iron and vitamin B12 by planning ahead or taking supplements. This way of eating is based on the idea that our hunter-gatherer ancestors ate a lot of whole, unprocessed foods like meat, fish, eggs, fruits, veggies, nuts, and seeds. It gets rid of processed foods, grains, and cheese.

Finding the Right Fit

Pay attention to how certain foods make you feel. Do you have more energy when you eat a lot of protein? Does adding more fiber make your gut feel better? Follow what your body tells you to do. Enjoy what nature has to offer! Try new fruits and vegetables to find healthy options you like and new flavors you like. Fats that are good for you are not bad! They are very important for making hormones, feeling full, and absorbing nutrients. Olive oil, nuts, seeds, avocado and avocado are all good sources of healthy fats. In the long run, strict diets may not work. Try to find a healthy, balanced diet that includes a wide range of tasty and nutritious foods. This lets you choose the items and the amount of food you eat. Try out new recipes and find ways to cook your food that are both healthy and tasty.

The Journey, Not the Destination. Wait, look into your choices, and don't be afraid to change how you do things along the way. The point is to find a way to eat that is good for your health and still lets you enjoy all the great foods that are out there. Be open to new experiences, try different flavors, and feed your body tasty, healthy foods. You might find that tasty treats are the way to a better you.

CHAPTER 4

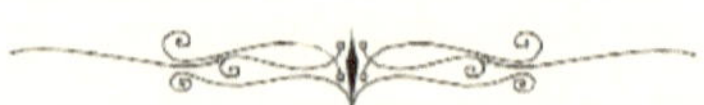

Conquering Cravings

"And Crushing Challenges"

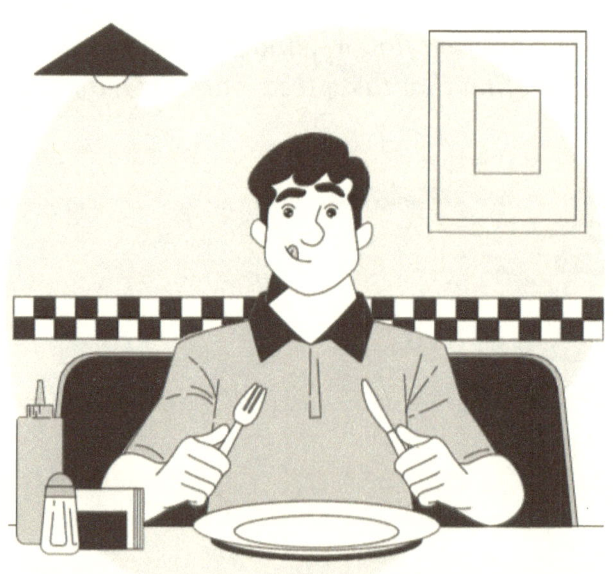

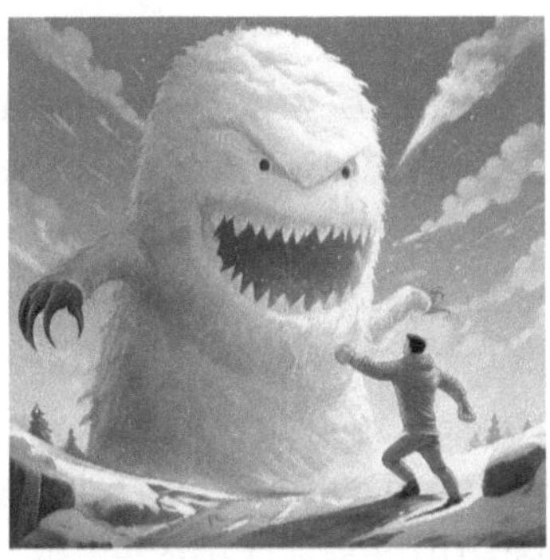

Outsmarting the Sugar Monster

*"Discover strategies to overcome cravings and
maintain a healthy relationship with food."*

Everyone has been there: the afternoon slump sets in, and the sweets start calling your name. Sugar cravings can be too strong, taking over your good goals and making you feel tired and guilty. Don't worry, sugar monster killer! You can beat your sweet tooth and have a good relationship with food if you know why you want certain foods and use some smart strategies.

Why Do We Want Sugar

If you eat a lot of processed foods and sugary drinks, your blood sugar levels will go up and down a lot. When blood sugar levels drop, people often want to eat sweets to get their energy back quickly. Our brains connect sugar to happiness. This link may make us crave that prize over time, even if it's not good for us. High amounts of the hormone cortisol can make you want sugary comfort foods when you're under a lot of stress. Cravings can sometimes be a sign of deeper problems, like being thirsty or not getting enough sleep. If you want to avoid sugar, pay attention to your body's cues and deal with the cause.

Tips to Get Around Cravings

Don't skip meals! Eat well-balanced meals and snacks all day to keep your blood sugar level steady and stop those cravings. To feel fuller for longer, eat healthy fats, lean protein, and complex carbs like whole grains. People often mistake being thirsty for being hungry. As the day goes on, drink a lot of water to stay hydrated and stop cravings that could be thirst hiding behind food. Know how to shop smart! Be careful of prepared foods that have extra sugar added to them. Choose foods that are naturally sweet and drink less sugary drinks. Do not let yourself get hangry! Keep healthy snacks like nuts and yogurt with berries and cut-up fruits and veggies on hand. This way, you'll always have a better choice on hand when you're hungry. Long-term worry can make you crave bad things. Try things like yoga, meditation, or deep breathing methods to help you deal with stress. When you don't get enough sleep, your body makes more of the hunger hormone ghrelin and less of the fullness hormone leptin. Aim for 7-8 hours of good sleep every night to keep your hormones in check and stop cravings. It can be bad to ban all sweets. Allow yourself small treats every once in a while. This keeps you from feeling deprived and encourages a good relationship with food. If you're craving something sweet, try something healthy. You could bake fruits with cinnamon, put berries in frozen yogurt, or use dark chocolate with at least 70% cacao. Fighting urges is only one part of the process. Mindful eating means taking your time to enjoy your food. Pay attention to when you feel hungry or full. Stop eating when you're full but not stuffed. The point of food is to enjoy it! Try out different tastes, textures, and ways of cooking. Take the time to enjoy and be aware of your meals. All things can be part of a healthy diet in small amounts. Don't worry about calling foods "good" or "bad." Instead, focus on eating healthily generally. Your body knows what's best for you. Pay attention to how different foods make you feel and choose foods that are good for your health and well-being as a whole.

You're not alone! Every once in a while, we all have urges. You can beat the sugar monster and take back control of your decisions if you understand why these things happen, use these strategies, and build a healthy relationship with food. Accept the process, be proud of your growth, and enjoy a life full of tasty, nutritious foods!

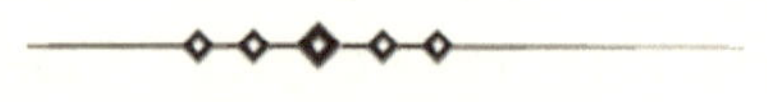

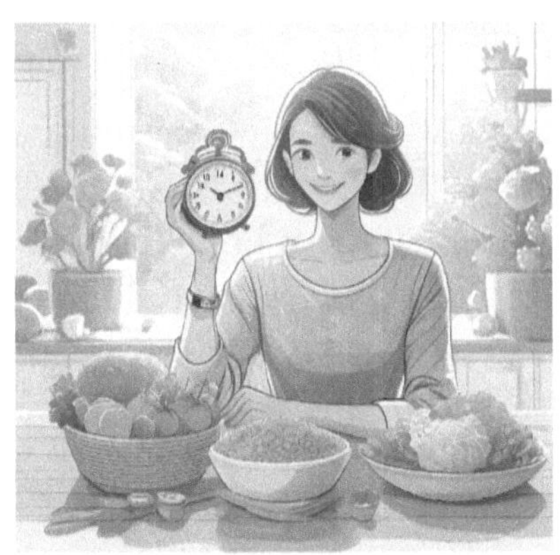

Time Management for Busy Healers

"Learn practical tips to prepare nourishing meals, even with a hectic schedule."

Being a counselor, like a doctor, nurse, therapist, or other health care worker, is a tough job. It can be hard to find time to eat well when you're working long hours, taking care of patients, and doing a lot of writing. Now for the good news: feeding your body healthy, tasty food doesn't have to take a lot of time. If you plan ahead and use a few smart tricks, you can feed your body well, even on busy days.

Take advantage of the power of planning.

Enjoy your weekends and plan your meals for the next week by setting aside a few hours on the weekends. This could mean looking at websites with healthy recipes, making a shopping plan, and preparing some ingredients ahead of time. Batch cooking is a great way to save time and money. You can make a lot of food on the weekend and then divide it up into servings for the week. You'll always have healthy meals ready to go, which will save you a lot of time during the week. Doing things ahead of time to save time, like chopping veggies, cooking grains, or marinating proteins, can save you a lot of time when you need it.

Quick and Healthy Meal Ideas

Chia seed overnight oats with berries and nuts are a great breakfast that you can grab and go. Either healthy egg cakes or Greek yogurt parfaits with granola and fruit can be made ahead of time and eaten quickly in the morning. Salads will save you time! Stock up on chopped and pre-washed veggies so you can make salads rapidly and in any way you like. For a healthy dinner, add protein like tofu, grilled chicken, or lentils. One great way to eat more veggies and protein is to make soups. On the weekend, make a big pot of lentil soup or minestrone. For lunch or dinner during the week, eat it. Sheet pan dinners are great! Put chopped meat, veggies, and spices on a sheet pan and season them. Bake it, and it's done! A healthy meal that doesn't take much time is ready. These are "The Mighty Leftovers." Do not forget how powerful leftovers can be! Make a bigger serving of a healthy dish for dinner, and the next day for lunch, eat what you saved.

Besides the Kitchen

Delivery services that bring you healthy meals can save you time. But if you choose this choice, watch out for portion sizes and sodium levels. To save time in the store, do your food shopping online or choose a pick-up option. This can help you avoid buying things you don't need and make your food shopping easier. It would help if you purchased a slow cooker because it works so well. Add the ingredients in the morning before work, and when you get home, you'll have a tasty and healthy meal ready to eat. Buy reusable containers. Preparing meals and putting them in reusable containers will make it easy to grab healthy foods on the go. Do not try to be great; instead, try to get better. You can make a big difference by making small changes, like eating more fruits and veggies or making healthy snacks ahead of time.

By using these tips and food ideas for managing your time, you can make sure that you don't forget to feed your body. A healer who is healthy and well-fed is a healer who works better, so taking care of yourself and your patients will benefit, too!

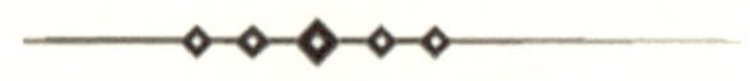

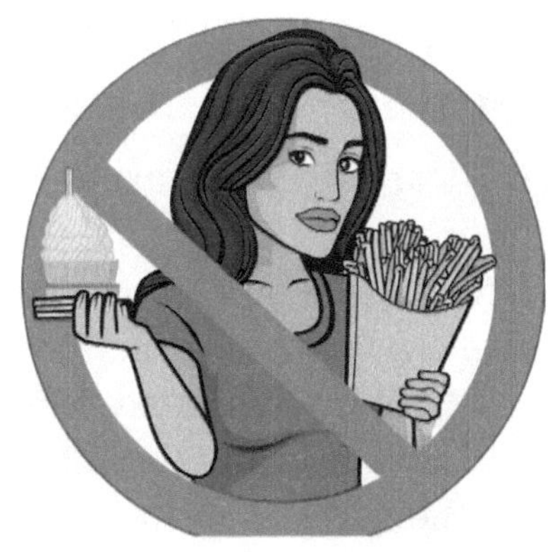

Building Resilience

"Navigating Social Gatherings and Travel"

At times, it can be hard to stick to healthy eating habits, especially when you're traveling or going to be with friends. Buffets, restaurant meals, and new places can make even the most serious health fanatic lose track. Don't worry, though! You can get through these situations without giving up your healthy lifestyle if you plan ahead and use a few tactics.

"Social Gatherings: How to Master the Art of Balance"

It's no secret that food is a big part of social events. Don't show up hungry! Before you leave, eat a healthy lunch. This makes you feel fuller, so you don't eat too much at the event. Choose smaller plates and try to enjoy every bite. Pacing yourself lets you enjoy the food and know when you're full before you eat too much. Choose healthy foods first. Before you eat something heavier, make sure your plate is full of fruits, veggies, and lean protein sources. You don't have to stay away from all the treats! Have a small amount of your favorite dessert or a treat from the area. The key is to indulge thoughtfully, not to deny your- self completely. People sometimes mistake thirst for hunger. During the event, drink water or tea without sugar to stay refreshed. This can also help you feel fuller for longer.

"Travel: Embracing Culinary Adventures Without Giving Up"

When you travel, you can learn about and experience new cultures, and food is often a big part of those. Learn about the food choices in the area before you go. Seek out places that serve healthy food that fits your dietary needs. Spend time in your local markets and pick out fresh fruits, veggies, and whole grains. This makes it possible to have meals that are both good and cheap. Look for places to stay that have kitchens. This gives you the freedom to cook some meals yourself, so you can always find healthy choices. When you eat out, choose smaller amounts and share your food with other travelers. In this way, you can try more kinds of things without eating too much. Choose fresh, local foods because they are usually less processed and better for you when you can. Ask how the food was cooked and choose grilled or steamed options. When you're on the go, bring healthy snacks like nuts, fruits, and breakfast bars. This keeps you from making bad choices at the vending machine or buying things at the store without thinking.

Building resilience: how you think is everything.

Keeping up good habits is all about getting stronger. Don't see trips or social events as obstacles. Instead, try to pick healthy options most of the time. A few treats now and then won't stop you from making progress. Pay attention to when you feel hungry or full. Don't feel like you have to finish everything you have in front of you. Don't stop eating until you're full. The point of food is to enjoy it! Enjoy the tastes, feelings, and people you're with. Don't just think about the calories; enjoy the event.

To keep a healthy lifestyle while going to parties and traveling, you need to plan ahead, make smart decisions, and be open to change. By being self-aware and planning ahead, you can enjoy new foods and social events with- out giving up your health and wellness goals. Get ready to see the world, one tasty and healthy bite at a time! Don't forget to bring your healthy attitude and your love of travel.

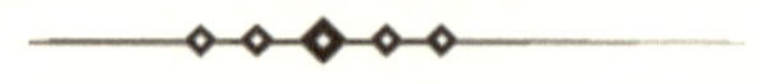

CHAPTER 5

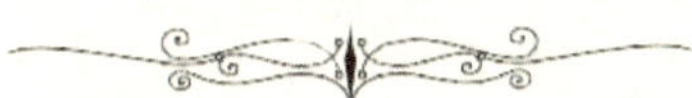

Mindful Munching

"Nourishing Body and Soul"

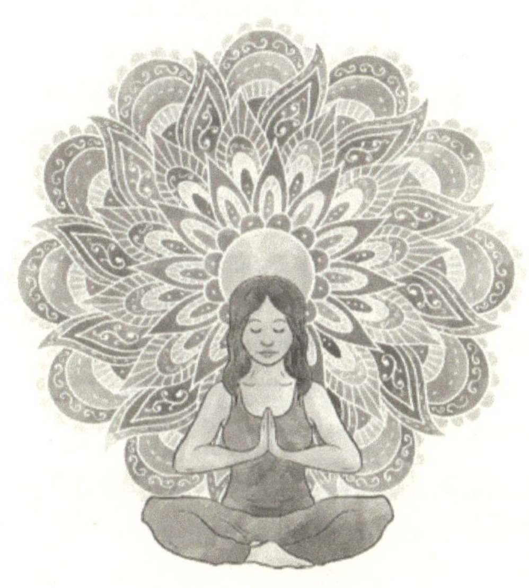

43

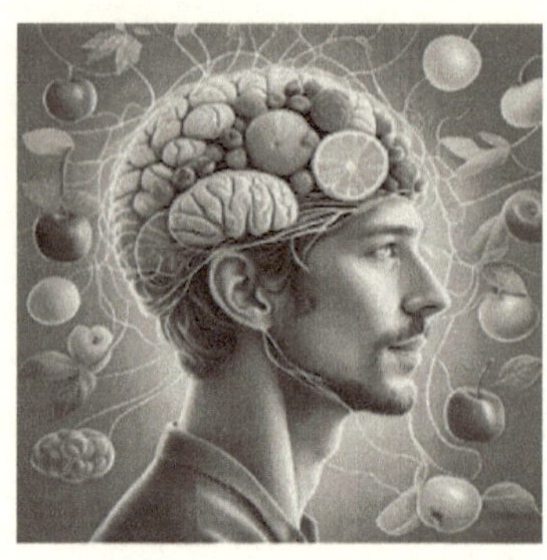

The Art of Mindful Eating

"Learn how to cultivate a mindful connection with food, savor each bite, and improve digestion."

People in our busy world often eat quickly, like taking a quick bite between meetings or mindlessly scrolling through social media while they pick at their food. But what if there was a way to make eating a mindful experience that not only gives your body what it needs but also makes you happy and makes digestion better? Let's learn how to eat properly. Mindful eating means becoming more aware of and appreciative of the food you eat. It's about taking your time, focusing on the present moment, and enjoying every bite. This practice has many benefits, such as better digestion, a happier relationship with food, and a greater sense of well-being. Setting up a space without any distractions is the first step to focused eating. Put down your phone, turn off the TV, and quiet any alerts. Focus on the food you're eating. Food is an event for the senses.

Spend a moment enjoying the looks, feels, and smells of your food before you eat it. This simple act of noticing can make you more excited and enjoy the experience more. Take little bites and really chew them. Enjoy how the food feels and tastes as it interacts with your taste buds. Take note of the subtleties like sweetness, saltiness, and softness that work together to make a one-of-a-kind taste experience. Mindful eating means paying attention to your body's signals for when it's hungry and when it's full. Take your time when you eat, and pay attention to how your body feels. Do you need more food after a few bites, or are you full? Do not push yourself to finish all the things you have to do. Listen to what your body is telling you. Mindful eating isn't about cutting back or not having what you want. It's about being aware and present while eating food. Let yourself enjoy all kinds of things, but be aware and purposeful about it.

The Good Things About Mindful Eating

If you eat slowly and chew each bite well, your body will be able to break down food more quickly, which will help you handle it better and absorb more nutrients. Mindful eating can help you pay attention to when you're hungry and stop yourself from eating too much. If you can recognize the signs of fullness, you'll be less likely to make bad decisions because you're eating without thinking. Eating mindfully can help you break free from emotional eating habits and build a healthier, more positive relationship with food. One benefit of slowing down and focusing on the present moment during a meal is that it can help lower stress and make you feel calm and healthy. Eating mindfully makes you respect all the work that goes into making food, from the farmer who grew the food to the person who cooked it.

Getting into the habit of mindful eating

"Start with One Meal" means to start by eating mindfully at one meal a day. Slowly add more meals to the routine until you feel comfortable with it. While you eat, pay attention to the present moment. Please pay attention to your feelings and thoughts without judging them, and then slowly bring your attention back to the act of eating. Learning to eat mindfully takes time and patience. Don't give up if you find yourself getting sidetracked at first. Just slowly turn your attention back to your food.

Mindful eating is a process, not a goal. More relationship with food, your body, and the present moment is what it's all about. You'll not only nourish your body with each mindful bite, but you'll also start living a more mindful and happy life.

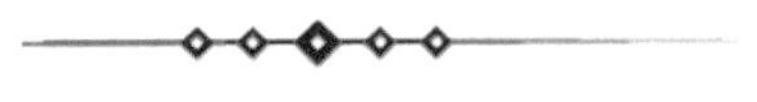

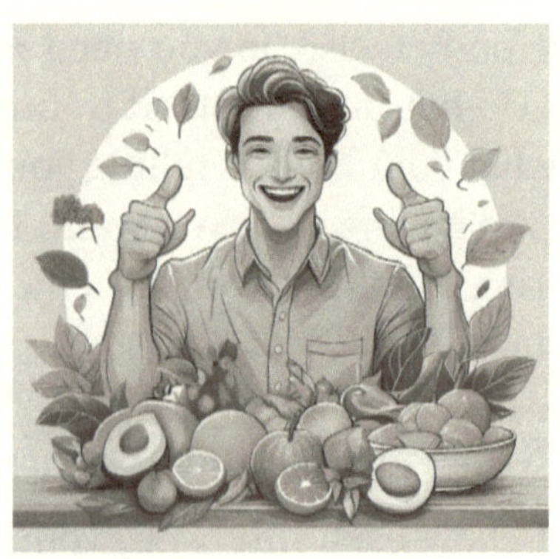

Taming the Inner Critic

"Develop self-compassion around food choices and focus on creating a positive relationship with eating."

We've all been there. As you reach for a cake slice, a voice inside your head says, "Bad choice!" "You'll feel bad about that later!" If you try to have a good relationship with food, this inner critic can get in the way. It will constantly judge the foods you choose, making you feel guilty and defeated. Self-compassion, on the other hand, can shut down the critic and help you become kinder and more sympathetic.

The Grip of the Inner Critic

The inner reviewer loves bad things. It tells you whether the foods you choose are "good" or "bad," which makes you feel bad and guilty. This kind of negativity can lead to a loop of not eating enough, cravings, and overeating.

Self-Compassion Saves the Day

Self-compassion is what you need to get rid of your inner judge. Kindness and understanding towards yourself are important, especially when you mess up with food. It means recognizing that everyone has trouble making food decisions sometimes, which is fine.

Pros of Self-Compassion

Being kind to yourself can help you deal with worry, which can make you eat poorly. Being nicer to yourself can help you feel less stressed about food and have a better relationship with it. Self-compassion makes you want to make good changes. If you are hard on yourself after failing, you will not want to try again as much. You're more likely to see mistakes as steps on your journey if you have self-compassion. Being kind to yourself helps you accept your flaws and all. This means recognizing that your relationship with food isn't perfect and focusing on growth instead of perfection. Being kind to yourself makes you more likely to eat mindfully. When you're nice to yourself, you're less likely to eat too much out of worry or guilt.

Tips for Being Kind to Yourself

Pay attention to the negative thoughts you have about the food you eat. What thoughts or words does your inner reviewer use? The first step to changing these habits is to become aware of them. Don't take the negative thoughts of your inner reviewer at face value. "Would I talk to a friend this way?" Replace bad thoughts with more positive ones. Everyone messes up with food sometimes. When you mess up, be kind to yourself. Allow yourself to forgive, learn from the mistake, and move on. Don't give up when things go wrong. No matter how small your growth is, be proud of it. Every decision you make with awareness is a step towards a better relationship with food. Don't judge your- self for the food you eat. Instead, ask yourself, "How does this food make me feel?" This makes you more aware of what your body needs and helps you make better choices.

Changing Your Attention

Do not think about "good" and "bad" things. Instead, think about how to have a good relationship with food. When you cook, you can control what goes into the food and how much you eat. Try out new, healthy meals until you find ones you like. Only eat when you're hungry and stop when you feel full. Please pay attention to when your body tells you it's hungry or full. Have fun at mealtimes! Enjoy the flavors, eat with people you care about, and be thankful for the nutrition that food gives you.

Learning to be kind to yourself and having a healthy relationship with food is a process, not a goal. You'll have some setbacks along the way, but with every mindful bite and act of self-kindness, your relationship with food will get better and more peaceful. Shut up your inner critic, show yourself kind- ness, and start a culinary adventure full of fun and discovery!

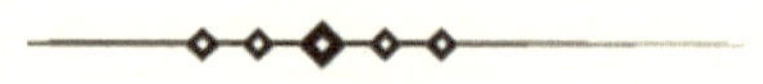

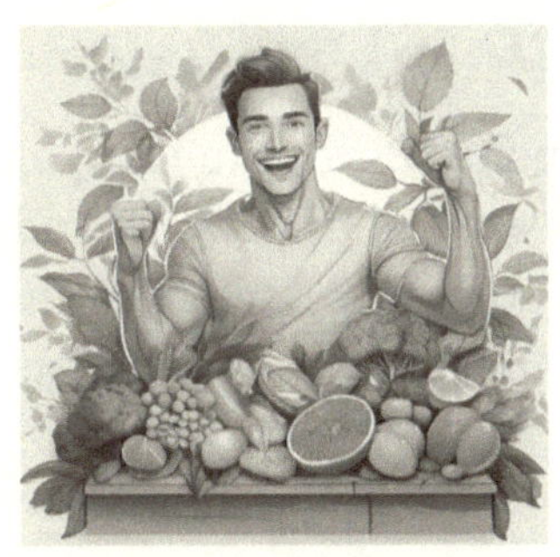

Food as a Celebration

"Explore ways to use mealtimes for connection, gratitude, and enjoyment."

Food gives our bodies what they need, but it has power that goes far beyond that. Food has always been an important part of celebrations, a way to connect with loved ones, show thanks, and make memories that will last a lifetime. Let's look at some ways to make mealtimes more than just a routine. Let's make them times of connection, joy, and happiness.

The Power of Sharing Plates

There's something special about eating with other people. It helps people feel like they are part of a group. Instead of individual plates, use family-style dishes or a potluck spread. This makes people more likely to talk, share stories, and feel like they are all in it together at the table.

Learn how to talk to people.

Put your phones down and turn off the TV! Mealtimes are great times to have really deep talks. When you share food with someone, ask them questions, listen to their stories, and get to know them. A meal with laughter, lively conversation, and touching moments is more fulfilling than a meal with silence.

Thank You Plates

By adding a "gratitude plate" to your meals, you can develop a mindset of gratitude. First, go around the table and say one thing you're thankful for. It can be something big or something small. This easy habit helps you value the food you have access to and the people who share it with you.

Themed Feasts

Get people excited and looking forward to things with special feasts! You can honor a cultural tradition, a favorite movie, or a special event by planning a meal with a theme. Decorate the table, make foods that go with the theme, and ask people to dress up for the party. These themed feasts make eating fun and memorable by letting people connect with each other.

Getting to know new people by breaking bread

Food can bring people together from different backgrounds. In between meals, use the time to meet new people. Have potlucks with co-workers, have neighbors over for dinner, or host nights with food from around the world. Sharing food helps people understand each other better, breaks down stereotypes, and makes friendships last.

Enjoying the Holidays and Traditions

Celebrate the wealth of each season by cooking with foods that are in season. Please find out about the traditional foods that are eaten during holidays or cultural events and make them with your family and friends. These food traditions help you feel like you belong, connect you to your history, and create memories that will last a lifetime.

The Pleasure of Cooking Slowly

It's important to slow down and enjoy the moment in our fast-paced world. Choose slow cookers or crockpots to make meals with little work. So, you can spend more time with your friends, setting the table and enjoying their company. Spend some time making a setting that looks good. Put out bright plates, cloth napkins, and fresh flowers on the table. A setup that looks good adds to the atmosphere and makes the meal more enjoyable. Make homemade meals for family members who are going through a hard time, new parents, or people who just need a pick-me-up to share the joy of food. Giving cooked food shows that you care, are warm, and support someone.

Celebrating with food doesn't have to cost a lot. It's about being deliberate and making a place for happiness, connection, and gratitude. By doing these simple things, you can turn meals into beautiful celebrations of life that you can share with loved ones and make memories that will last a lifetime. We should all break bread together, enjoy the flavors, and celebrate how food can bring people together!

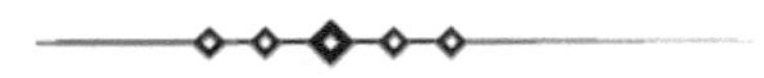

CHAPTER 6

Move Your Body

"Heal Your Soul: Yoga's Role in Recovery"

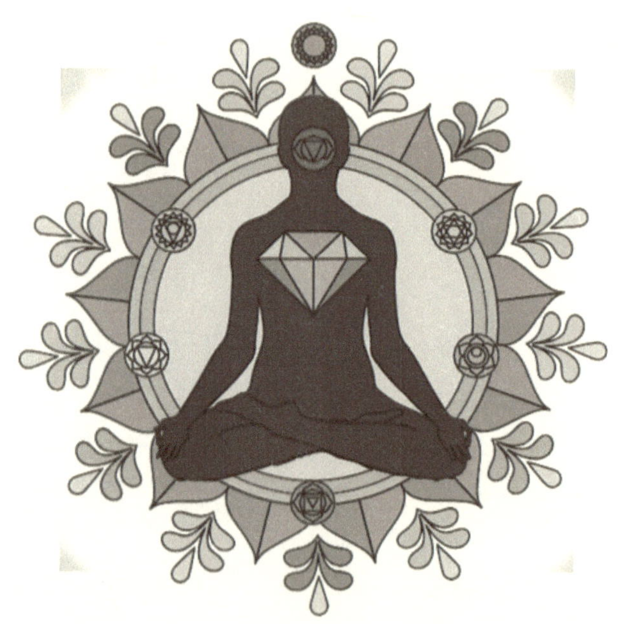

Yoga: A Journey of Body and Mind

"Discover the powerful synergy between gentle yoga practices and the healing process."

Are you experiencing a sense of exhaustion? Looking to recover from an accident or simply find a way to improve your overall health and well-being? There is no better option than yoga! Through the use of gentle movements and the healing process, this age-old practice creates a powerful synergy that promotes harmony for both the body and the mind. The entire approach that yoga takes is where its charm lies. Hatha yoga, often known as gentle postures, places an emphasis on conscious movements and lengthening of the body. In addition to enhancing flexibility and strengthening muscles, these poses also promote circulation, all of which can contribute to the healing and recuperation process. Yet yoga is not limited to the physical realm. The longer you hold these pos- es, the more you will notice that your breathing will automatically slow down. By practicing pranayama, also known as mindful breathing, one can better manage stress and anxiety, both of which can frequently impede the healing process. The practice of yoga produces an ideal atmosphere for your body to concentrate on recuperation since it makes the mind more at ease and encourages relaxation. The advantages are not limited to that. Yoga fosters a greater awareness of oneself. As you progress through the positions, you will become more aware of the feelings that are occurring within your body. Because of this awareness, you can recognize regions that may require additional care or attention during the process of healing.

Yoga is a beautiful practice since it is so easy to practice. Since gentle yoga activities are appropriate for people of all fitness levels, they are an ideal supplement to any rehabilitation process. Yoga is a gentle yet powerful way to support your body and mind, and it can be beneficial for a variety of reasons, including the management of chronic pain, recovery from an injury, or just the pursuit of a road to greater well-being. To begin your journey towards healing via the mindful movements of yoga, roll out your mat, take a deep breath, and get ready to go on a journey.

Stress Reduction Through Movement

"Learn simple yoga postures to promote relaxation, manage stress, and enhance sleep."

In a state of being overpowered by stress? Are you having trouble sleeping at night? The power of movement is not something to be underestimated! Certain yoga postures have the potential to be a game-changer for reducing stress, improving sleep quality, and improving general well-being. The following are some positions that are more suitable for beginners and can be incorporated into your everyday routine:

Balasana, also known as Child's Pose

When you've had a long day, this relaxing stance is a wonderful way to decompress and relax. Your forehead should be resting on the ground when you are kneeling on the floor and sitting back on your heels. Your palms should be facing down when you extend your arms out in front of you. Inhale deeply and maintain the pose for a number of breaths, allowing your body to get completely immersed in the position.

Marjaryasana-Bitilasana, also known as the Cat-Cow Pose

By performing this sequence of mild movements, you will stretch and strengthen your spine. On all fours, with your hands shoulder-width apart and your knees hip-width apart, begin the exercise. While you are inhaling, make a cow position by arching your back and looking up. You should assume the cat stance by rounding your back and bringing your chin to your chest as you exhale. Your breath should flow between these movements, and you should repeat this process multiple times.

Known as Adho Mukha Svanasana

Downward-Facing Dog is a yoga pose. To enhance circulation, this time-honored stance helps to quiet the mind. Beginning on all fours, thrust your hips back and up while simultaneously straightening your legs to the greatest extent that is comfortable for you. Maintain a position in which your head is in line with your arms and your heels are pressing toward the floor. Continue to hold for a few breaths.

Corporeal Pose, also known as Savasana

You can completely relax your body by adopting this restorative stance. With your arms at your sides and your palms facing upward, lie down on your back in a flat position. Keep your eyes closed and concentrate on your breathing. Put an end to any tension you may be experiencing and just be for a few minutes.

The Bridge Pose, also known as Setu Bandhasana:

Stretching your chest and opening your hips are two benefits of this easy back-bend. If you are lying on your back, bend your knees and place your feet flat on the ground. To create a straight line from your knees to your shoulders, lift your hips off the ground and create a straight line. As a means of providing support, interlace your fingers under your torso. Continue to hold for a few breaths.

Maintaining consistency is essential! Make it a goal to practice these positions every day, even if it's just for a few minutes. You can experiment with other positions as you feel more comfortable, or you could consider enrolling in a yoga class that is designed for beginners. It will come as a surprise to you how these straightforward movements may alleviate tension, enhance the quality of your sleep, and leave you feeling revitalized and refreshed if you engage in them with determination.

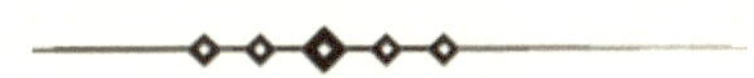

Yoga for All Bodies

"Explore yoga modifications to make the practice accessible and enjoyable for every individual."

Even while yoga is frequently depicted as a practice that is reserved for those who are youthful and flexible, the reality is that yoga is for everyone! The flexibility of yoga is one of its most attractive features. It is possible to make even the most fundamental poses accessible and pleasant for people of all body types by making a few straightforward adjustments.

Embrace Props

Don't let your physical limitations prevent you from achieving your goals! When practicing yoga, you may find that props such as blocks, straps, and bolsters are your greatest friends. It is possible to lift your hands in poses such as Downward-Facing Dog by using blocks, which makes these postures more ac- accessible for individuals who have tension in their hamstrings. The use of straps can assist you in lengthening and deepening stretches, while the use of bolsters can provide support and comfort when adopting restorative positions. Please pay attention to your body. The practice of yoga does not involve forcing oneself into uncomfortable poses. Self-discovery and awareness of one's body are the goals of this voyage. If a particular stance causes you discomfort, don't be afraid to adjust it! It is always possible to find an alternative that provides comparable advantages without causing discomfort.

Put your attention on alignment rather than perfection

Don't let yourself become preoccupied with striking the "perfect" pose that is portrayed in photographs. The way you do yoga is a reflection of your body. Concentrate on keeping a comfortable position and ensuring that you are properly aligned.

Various Downward-Facing Dog Variations

It is possible to adapt this traditional position to meet a variety of challenges. It is recommended that you try a "dolphin pose" if you have tight hamstrings. This pose involves maintaining your forearms on the ground while elevating your hips slightly. Consider adopting a "puppy pose" for those who are having problems with their lower back. In this pose, you will rest your forehead on the ground while extending your arms forward.

Warriors Pose with Support

Warrior poses are particularly beneficial for strengthening the legs, but they can be difficult to perform for individuals who have knee problems. Take advantage of a chair as a support. Instead of stretching your hand back, you should rest it on the back of the chair in Warrior II so that you can maintain your equilibrium.

Pose variations that are performed when seated

Seating oneself in a chair allows for the practice of a variety of yoga poses. This is an excellent choice for people who have limited movement or who have sustained injuries. While seated in a comfortable position, you can perform abdominal twists, forward bends, and even arm stretches.

Practicing yoga is more of a journey than a destination. Embrace changes, pay attention to what your body is telling you, and concentrate on the pleasure of movement. Regardless of the physical constraints you may have, there is a yoga practice that is suitable for you, and with a little bit of imagination, you may unlock the transformational power of yoga.

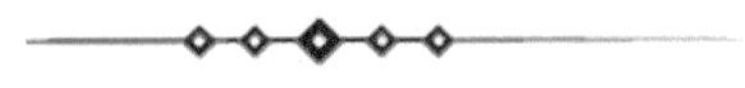

CHAPTER 7

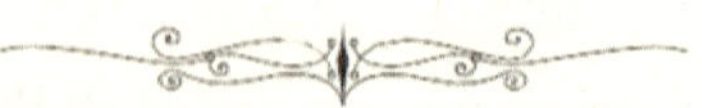

Nature's Bounty

"Superfoods for Recovery"

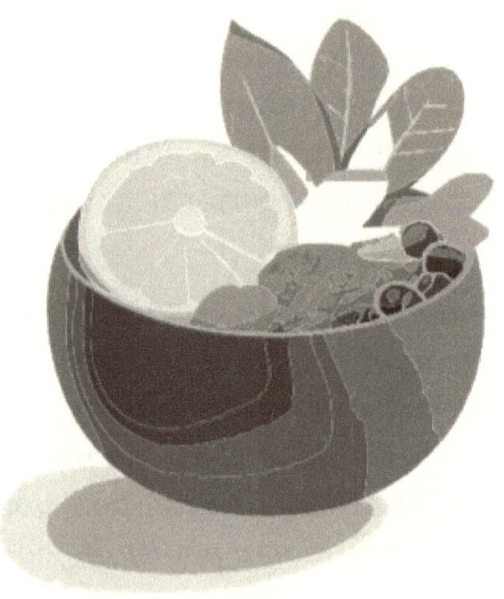

Unlocking the Power of Plants

*"Discover a variety of nutrient-rich superfoods
that can accelerate your healing journey."*

Our bodies are amazing machines that can fix us in amazing ways. But sometimes, it helps a lot to have a little extra help. Welcome to the world of plant-based superfoods, which are nutrient-dense powerhouses that can help you heal faster and give your body more energy.

The Allure of Superfoods

Superfoods aren't just a way to make money. They are full of vitamins, minerals, antioxidants, phytonutrients, and other good things for your body that it needs to stay healthy. A lot of health problems are linked to chronic inflammation. Berries and leafy veggies are two superfoods that are high in antioxidants and can help fight inflammation and improve your health in general. To make your immune system stronger, Your immune system is the first line of defense against getting sick. Foods that are high in beta-carotene (found in sweet potatoes and carrots) and vitamin C (found in bell peppers and citrus fruits) can help your immune system.

Help with detoxification

Our bodies naturally clean themselves out, but sometimes they need some extra help. A lot of chlorophyll can help your body get rid of toxins. Superfoods like broccoli, Brussels sprouts, and chlorella are full of it. In the mending process, some superfoods can help in certain ways. For example, bone broth has a lot of collagen which helps keep muscles and joints healthy.

Exploring the Kingdom of Superfoods

Berries are full of fiber and antioxidants, making them a great food choice. They're great fresh, frozen, or mixed into drinks. Leafy greens like kale, spinach, and Swiss chard are full of enzymes, vitamins, and minerals. You can blend them into green drinks or put them in salads or stir-fries. Some foods that are good for you and help reduce inflammation are broccoli, cauliflower, Brussels sprouts, and cabbage. You can roast them, steam them, or put them in stews and soups. This colorful root vegetable has a lot of beta-carotene, which helps keep your eyes and immune system healthy. You can roast them, mash them, or bake them into fries. This soup is full of collagen, which helps keep your joints and gut healthy. For a healthy homemade broth, simmer bones with veggies and herbs. This root can be used in many ways and is good for digestion and reducing inflammation. For a soothing drink, you can mix it into drinks or stir-fries. Garlic is said to help your defense system and give your food a tasty kick.

Take it raw, roast it, or sauté it. The golden spice can help with pain and inflammation. You can put it in soups, stews, or golden milk lattes. The great thing about superfoods is that they work together. When you mix different kinds, you get a powerful nutritional punch. For instance, eat bell peppers with fresh greens that are high in vitamin C to get even more vitamin C. You can get more Superfood Power than just what you eat: You can also take care of yourself by eating superfoods. Antioxidants are found in large amounts in green tea, and aloe vera can be used to soothe itchy skin.

Superfoods are a great way to add variety and balance to your diet. Don't get too excited about just one vitamin. It is important to eat a range of these healthy plants at meals and snacks. Let the colorful world of superfoods be your guide as you start to heal. They will give your body the power of nature.

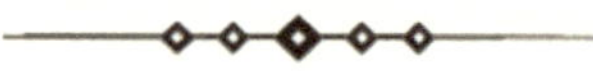

From Seed to Superpower

"Explore the unique benefits of specific superfoods like berries, leafy greens, and adaptogenic herbs."

There are many powerful foods in nature. Some of them are called "super-foods" because they have a lot of good nutrients in a small amount of space. In addition to providing food, these plant-based powerhouses offer a wide range of health benefits. Now that we know what superfoods are let's look at the benefits of berries, leafy veggies, and adaptogenic herbs. There are a lot of antioxidants in "The Berry Bunch." Berries are like little blasts of color and flavor, but what makes them special is that they have a lot of antioxidants. These strong molecules fight free radicals, which are unstable molecules that hurt cells and cause many health problems. These little blue gems are great for your brain. Studies show that they might help your brain and mind work better. Berries are full of vitamin C and antioxidants, which can help your defense system and reduce swelling. Cranberries and sour berries are good for your urinary tract and may even help keep you from getting UTIs. Goji berries are an important part of traditional Chinese medicine because they are full of antioxidants and immune-boosting polysaccharides. They are also thought to be good for your general health.

Leafy green giants are food powerhouses that are full of important nutrients. Don't forget about the humble growing green! Because they are so high in fiber, vitamins, and minerals, these foods are essential to a healthy diet. This popular green is a great way to get vitamin K, which is important for healthy bones and blood clotting. It has a lot of fiber and vitamins as well. Spinach said, "Popeye knew what he was doing!" Spinach is a great way to get iron, which is needed for the body to carry air. Plus, it has vitamins A and C. Swiss Chard green vegetables are very useful. It has a lot of magnesium, which helps muscles and nerves work, and vitamins A, C, and K. What are collard greens? These hearty greens have a lot of calcium, which is good for teeth and bones. They also have a lot of vitamins A, C, and K. Adaptogenic herbs are nature's way of making you stronger. Adaptogenic herbs are a special group of plants that help the body deal with stress. These powerhouses can help you relax, give you more energy, and make you healthier overall. This old Indian plant is called an "adaptogen" because it helps the body deal with worry and anxiety. It might also help you sleep better. This adaptogenic plant has been shown to make people less stressed and tired. It may also help them concentrate and perform better physically. This superfood from Peru has been used for a long time to give people more energy and strength. It may also help keep hormones healthy. It is known that this holy herb can help people adjust. It might help your brain work better, give you more energy, and keep your defense system strong.

How to Unlock the Synergy

The real magic of superfoods is how they work together. When you mix different kinds, you get a powerful nutritional punch. For instance, to get more vitamin C, eat bell peppers with fresh greens that are high in vitamin C. Do not be afraid to try new things and make colorful, superfood-rich meals!

Power of Superfoods Beyond the Plate

Superfoods are good for you in more ways than one. Aloe vera can be put on sensitive skin to make it feel better, and green tea, which is full of antioxidants, can be drunk as a healthy and refreshing drink.

It would help if you thought of superfoods as an addition to a healthy, varied diet. Choose a whole-food approach that includes a wide range of fruits, veggies, and whole grains to get the most out of plant-based nutrition. As you learn more about superfoods, keep in mind that these little powerhouses can help you get to the best health and well-being possible.

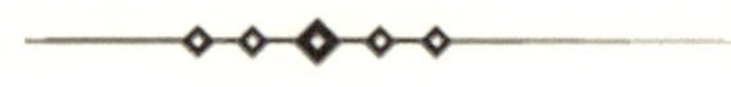

Incorporating Superfoods

Even though the word "superfood" sounds scary, adding them to your diet doesn't have to be hard. The key is to come up with fun and tasty ways to sneak these healthy foods into your daily meals and snacks. Let's look at some easy and delicious ways to make your food stronger!

Breakfast Boost

Get a boost of vitamins to start the day! Put a big amount, of blueberries, raspberries, or strawberries on top of your yogurt or muesli in the morning. They're so healthy and refreshing that you can even put them in your drink. Make your drink eco-friendly! For a nutritious breakfast on the go, blend spinach or kale with your favorite vegetables, yogurt, and a splash of plant-based milk. Chia seeds are very healthy because they are full of fiber and omega-3 fatty acids. For extra health benefits, sprinkle them on top of your yogurt, rice, cereal, or other foods.

Power-Up for Lunch

Make your salad sound like an orchestra of healthy foods! Chop up some kale, spinach, or Swiss chard and add it to the base for a healthy diet. Don't forget to add some avocado pieces for a creamy taste and healthy fats. Add a lot of vegetables to your lunch with soup. If you want a healthy and comforting meal, roast some veggies like broccoli, cauliflower, and sweet potatoes and then blend them with your favorite broth. Plus, points if you add some Greek yogurt for nutrition.

Eating Smart Snacks

Instead of a sugary trail mix, make your superfood mix for a healthy and filling snack: mixed nuts, seeds (like sunflower or pumpkin seeds), and dried fruits (like cranberries or goji berries). Edamame, which is a young soybean, is a great way to get protein and fiber from plants. They are already cooked inside the pod, which makes them a great snack to take with you. Making guacamole is a tasty way to use avocado's healthy fats. For a healthy and filling lunch, eat it with whole-wheat crackers or vegetable sticks.

Delightful Dinner

Want to sneak some superfoods into your dinner? You can chop up zucchini or cauliflower rice and mix it with ground meat to make burgers, meatballs, or even lasagna. You won't even notice the extra vegetables, but your body will thank you! Healthy omega-3 fatty acids can be found in large amounts in salmon. Cooked Brussels sprouts and sweet potatoes make a full, tasty meal that is full of superfoods. Lentils are a cheap superfood that is high in fiber and protein. Make a rich soup or stew with them for a warm and healthy meal.

Being consistent is very important! You can make your diet healthier and tastier without making big changes to your schedule by creating these simple swaps, which add to your daily routine. So, let your cooking imagination run wild and start an adventure exploring superfoods!

CHAPTER 8

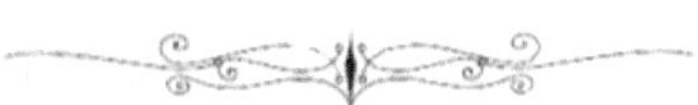

Navigating the Supplement Sea

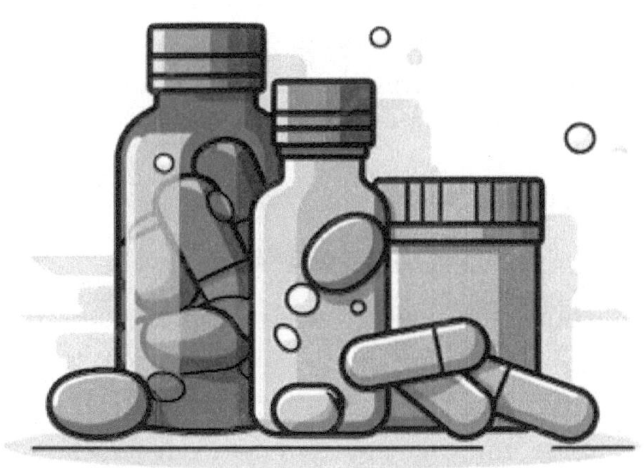

Demystifying Supplements:

"Understand the different types of supplements and how they can support your recovery goals."

When you go to the store, have you ever felt like there were too many supplements to choose from? There were rows and rows of bottles with labels that were hard to understand. The labels promised everything from stronger muscles to glowing skin. Do not be afraid, health explorer! This guide will help you find your way around the world of supplements and figure out how they might help you reach your healing goals.

To begin, it's important to note that supplements are not magic bullets.

Supplements do exactly what they sound like they do—they add to a healthy food and way of life. They're not a one-size-fits-all answer; think of them as ex-people on your health team. Foods that are good for you, like fruits, vegetables, whole grains, and lean protein, should always be the basis of your health. Supplements can then be thought of to make up for any possible food gaps or support specific needs.

Learning About the Different Kinds of Supplements:

These are important chemicals that our bodies need to work right. A multivitamin can help you make sure you're getting the daily recommended amount of minerals and vitamins, especially if you think you might be missing some in your food. These are protein powders popular with players and people who want to get stronger. Protein is important for building and repairing muscles, and you can get a lot of it from whole foods like fish, lean meats, and beans. If it's hard for you to get enough protein from food alone or after a workout, protein powder might be a good choice. This is about omega-3 fatty acids. These good fats are important for keeping your heart healthy, keeping your brain working well, and lowering inflammation. For people who don't eat enough fish, pills can be a good alternative. Fatty fish- like salmon and tuna are great sources. The good bacteria in your gut are a lot like these live bacteria. They help keep your gut healthy and your digestion working well, which is good for your general health. Probiotics are found in fermented foods like kimchi and yogurt, or you can take them in pill form. Supplements with herbs. This group includes a lot of different plant-based products, each of which is said to have health benefits. Turmeric, which is known to reduce inflammation, and ashwagandha, which is an adaptogen that may help you deal with stress, are two well-known examples. Before taking any herbal supplement, it's import- ant to do your research and talk to a doctor or nurse because it might interact with other medicines or cause side effects.

Choosing supplements that help you reach your recovery goals

Cells can heal with the help of supplements like vitamin C, zinc, and protein. For personalized advice based on your unique injury, talk to a medical professional. Protein, some vitamins, and minerals, and getting better after an accident may be very important for wound healing and tissue repair. Because of your surgery, your doctor will probably tell you to take certain vitamins. If you feel tired or think you might not be getting enough of certain nutrients, a multivitamin or specific supplements like vitamin D or iron (based on blood tests) can help fill in the gaps and improve your health as a whole.

Important Things to Think About Before Supplementing

Always talk to your doctor: Before taking any supplement, speak to your doctor or nurse about it. They can tell you about possible interactions between the vitamins and medicines you are already taking and make sure they are safe and right for your needs. Pick names that are known for having high standards for quality control. Check for signs of approval from outside groups, such as the USP (United States Pharmacopoeia) or NSF International. It's not always better to have more. To avoid possible side effects, it is very important to follow the dose instructions on the bottle. Notice how you feel after taking a vitamin. If the product makes you feel bad, stop using it and talk to your doctor.

Supplements might help you get better, but they should never be used instead of a healthy food and way of life. For best health, put eating whole foods, regular exercise, and enough sleep at the top of your list. You can find supplements that might help you get better with a little study, some advice from your doctor, and a healthy dose of skepticism.

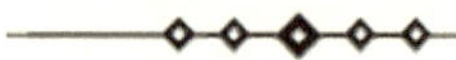

Quality Over Quantity

*"Learn how to choose high-quality supplements
and avoid unnecessary ones."*

It can be hard to know where to start with supplements. Because there are so many bottles that claim to be the cure-all, it's easy to believe the hype and buy more than you need. But keep in mind that quality is more important than number when it comes to supplements. Here's how to find your way around the aisle and pick out good supplements while dodging ones you don't need:

Pay attention to food first.

Supplements should not be used instead of a healthy diet, but rather to add to it. A wholesome meal full of fruits, vegetables, whole grains, and lean protein should be your top priority. Making sure your body gets the nutrients it needs from natural sources is important.

Figure out what you need.

It's not cool to take a vitamin. Think about it:

- ✓ "Do I have any diagnosed deficiencies?" A blood test can tell you if you're missing a certain mineral or vitamin.

- ✓ "Do I have any specific health goals I'm aiming for?" Some, products, like protein powder for building muscle or omega-3s for heart health, may help in specific ways.

- ✓ Do I have any food allergies? People who are vegetarians or vegans might benefit from taking iron or vitamin B12 pills.

Talk to your doctor

Talk to your doctor before taking any supplements because supplements can mix with some conditions or medicines. Get advice on the right doses Because too much of a good thing can be bad. Based on your specific needs, your doctor can tell you what dose is safe and helpful for you. Help you figure out which supplements you don't need; they may find that the nutrients you get from food are enough for you.

Quality Is Important

Choose names that are known for maintaining high-quality standards. Look for certifications from outside groups such as USP (United States Pharmacopeia) or NSF International. These make sure that the vitamin meets quality standards. Please pay attention to the amount, the chemicals, and any allergens that might be in it. Look for pills that don't have any fillers, additives, or fake ingredients that you don't need.

Less is More

Try not to take too many pills at once. Pay attention to your special needs, and don't forget that a healthy, well-balanced diet is the most important thing for your health. Pay attention to how you feel after taking a vitamin. If it makes you feel bad, like having stomach problems or headaches, stop taking it and talk to your doctor.

Please do not believe the marketing hype.

Flashy packaging and recommendations from famous people don't always mean the product is good. When making decisions, do your homework and pay attention to trusted names and scientific proof.

Adopt a holistic approach.

Don't forget that vitamins are only one part of the picture. For the best health, make a balanced diet, regular exercise, getting enough sleep, and learning how to deal with stress a top priority. These tips will help you feel more confident as you explore the world of supplements. For a more complete approach to your health, choose quality over number, talk to your doctor, and put whole foods first.

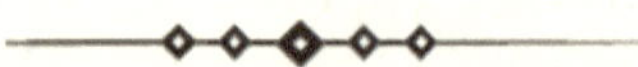

Partnering with a Healthcare Professional

"Discover the importance of working with a healthcare professional to develop a personalized supplement plan."

Supplements can be hard to understand because there are so many aisles, labels, and claims. Some say they can fix everything, while others may not help much or even be harmful to your health. This is where a healthcare worker (HCP) can help you. To make a supplement plan that is safe, successful, and fits your needs, you need to work with a doctor, registered dietitian, or other qualified health care professional (HCP).

Why work with an HCP?

HCPs know enough about vitamins to figure out how they work scientifically. They can help you tell the difference between fact and myth and find supplements that have a strong scientific basis for the health benefits they claim to offer. Blood tests can show nutritional gaps that were not known to be there. Your primary care doctor (HCP) can help you understand these data and suggest specific supplements to fill in any nutritional gaps. When you take certain vitamins with medicines you're already on, they might not work as well or cause side effects-you don't want. Your HCP can look at possible conflicts and make sure that your supplement plan is safe and won't affect the way your other medicines work. Supplement labels often list a range of doses that are thought to be safe. Your healthcare provider (HCP) can change the dose based on your needs, age, and overall health. With vitamins, there is no "one size fits all" method. Your HCP can make a personalized plan for you by looking at your health goals, your habits, and any health conditions you already have.

What to Talk About with Your HCP

Talk about your medical background, including any medicines you're taking and any health problems you already have. Be honest about what you eat. This will help your HCP figure out what nutrition gaps you might have that supplements can fill. Do you want to improve your athletic ability, your immune system, or a specific deficiency? By telling your HCP your goals, they can make better suggestions for you.

Building a Relationship for Working Together

It's okay to ask questions. Don't be afraid to ask your HCP why they think you should take certain vitamins and what side effects might happen. Your HCP can help you more if you tell them more about your health and how you live.

You can make a safe and effective supplement plan that helps your general health journey if you work together. Now that you know you have a trained professional by your side, you can go into the supplement aisle without being confused.

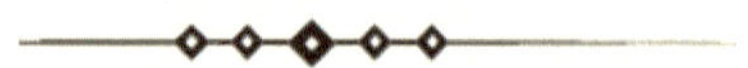

CHAPTER 9

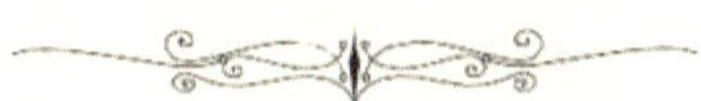

Food for Thought

"Nutritional Pathways to a Brighter Mindset"

The Brain-Gut Connection

"Explore how gut health impacts your mood, focus, and overall mental well-being."

For many years, the gut was thought of as the body's plumbing system, working to digest food and get rid of trash. However, new research has found an interesting and complicated way for the gut and brain to talk to each other. This is called the gut-brain link. This complex connection shows how the health of our gut microbiome—the trillions of bacteria that live in our digestive system—can have a big effect on our mood, ability to concentrate, and general mental health.

The gut microbiome is like an orchestra made of tiny organisms.

Think about a busy city inside your gut. The gut microbiome is a complex environment made up of trillions of bacteria, fungi, and other microbes. These tiny residents are very important for many body processes, such as digestion, nutrient absorption, and immune system control. But they affect more than just our guts; they also affect our minds through a complex web of communication pathways.

The Vagus Nerve: The Road Between the Gut and the Brain

The main way that the gut and brain talk to each other is through the vagus nerve. This long, winding nerve sends and receives messages between the two organs all the time. The gut microbiome sends calming messages through the vagus nerve when it is healthy and balanced. This makes you feel good and relaxed. On the other hand, an unbalanced gut microbiome can cause stress signals that can cause sadness, anxiety, and even brain fog.

What Gut Health Has to Do with Mental Health: The Power of Microbes

The gut bacteria not only talk to the brain but also play a big part in creating neurotransmitters, which are chemicals that control mood, sleep, and thinking.

Neurotransmitters, such as serotonin, also known as the "feel-good" hormone, are made by good bacteria in the gut. A healthy; bacteria make sure that your body makes enough serotonin, which makes you feel good and happy. On the other hand, an unbalanced gut microbiome can stop serotonin production, which could cause sadness and anxiety. Brain-derived neurotrophic factor (BDNF) is a protein that is important for learning, memory, and brain function. The gut helps make BDNF. Studies show that a healthy gut microbiome can help the body make more BDNF, which can improve cognitive ability and focus. On the other hand, an unbalanced gut bacteria may lead to memory loss and brain fog. The bacteria in the gut have a big effect on how the body reacts to stress. When you're stressed, your gut makes chemicals like cortisol. A good microbiome, on the other hand, can help keep cortisol levels in check, which can make you feel calm and strong. On the other hand, a bad gut can make the stress reaction worse, which can cause anxiety and make it hard to handle stress.

What You Eat Can Change Your Mood: Feeding Your Gut and Mind

The bacteria in our gut are directly affected by what we eat. Prebiotics are fibers that your body can't break down. They feed the good bugs in your gut. There are live bacteria in probiotics that help keep your gut microbiome healthy and diverse. You can take care of your gut microbiome by eating fermented foods like yogurt and kimchi and fruits, veggies, and whole grains that are high in prebiotics. Too much sugar and processed foods can make dangerous bacteria grow in the gut, which can throw off the microbiome's delicate balance. This can cause inflammation, which can make you feel bad and make it hard to think clearly. It's good for your gut to eat slowly, enjoy your food, and keep your stress under control while you eat.

"Beyond Diet: Supporting the Link Between Your Gut and Brain"

A healthy gut microbiome is supported by regular physical exercise. Aim to work out at a reasonable level for at least 30 minutes most days of the week. Getting enough sleep is important for your gut health and your general health. Aim to get at least 7-8 hours of good sleep every night. The gut microbiome can be messed up by long-term worry. To keep your gut healthy, do things that help you relax, like yoga, meditation, or deep breathing.

The Future of the Brain-Gut Link

The area of studying the link between the gut and the brain is changing very quickly. Researchers are looking into how changing the gut microbiome might help treat a wide range of mental illnesses, from Alzheimer's disease and anxiety to sadness and fear. Even though more studies need to be done, in the future, traditional therapies and strategies that target the gut microbiome may be used.

Nourishing Your Neurotransmitters

"Learn how specific foods can support the production of mood-boosting brain chemicals."

Have you ever thought about why one tasty meal can make you happy and energized while another makes you tired and cranky? The answer is in your brain, in the complex dance of neurotransmitters. Neurotransmitters are chemical signals that control your mood, sleep, focus, and health in general. The good news? Your food choices can change this dance! You can help your body make more of these mood-boosting neurotransmitters by eating certain foods that are high in certain nutrients. This will naturally make you happy and healthier.

The Orchestra of Neurotransmitters

Neurotransmitters are like the players in your brain, which is like a busy concert hall. Each neurotransmitter affects different parts of your brain state in its own way. Also known as the "happy hormone," serotonin controls your mood, sleep, and hunger. Having low amounts of serotonin can make you depressed, anxious, or have trouble sleeping. In the brain, this neurotransmitter is linked to happiness, motivation, and rewards. It is very important for learning, moving, and focusing. People who don't get enough dopamine can feel sluggish, lose drive, and have trouble concentrating. While this neurotransmitter calms the nervous system and makes you feel good, it also makes you feel peaceful. Low amounts of GABA can make it harder to sleep and cause anxiety. This ex-citatory chemical is very important for memory, learning, and brain function. Too much glutamate, on the other hand, can be bad and cause worry and brain fog.

"Food as a Conductor: Orchestrating the Production of Neurotransmitters"

Good news: your food can change how many of these neurotransmitters your body makes. These foods can help you feel good by coordinating a musical score of good chemicals in your brain:

Symphony of Serotonin

This amino acid is a building block for serotonin. Turkey, chicken, fish, eggs, and dairy items should all be part of your diet. Complex carbs, which can be found in whole grains, sweet potatoes, and fruits, keep blood sugar levels balanced, which is needed to make serotonin. This vitamin is required in order to turn tryptophan into serotonin. Eat foods like potatoes, beans, and bananas.

Dopamine Duets:

Dopamine is made with the help of another amino acid called tyrosine. Eat foods like chicken, fish, beans, and lentils that are high in protein. A cofactor for enzymes that help make dopamine is this mineral. Leafy greens, red meat, and beans are all iron-rich foods that you should eat. Omega-3 fatty acids are found in flaxseeds, fatty fish like; salmon and tuna, and other foods. They help the brain make dopamine and other chemicals that control mood.

GABA's Soft Lullaby

Glutamate is important for brain activity, but too much of it can be bad. To keep things in balance, eat less prepared foods and MSG, which are high in free glutamate. Yogurt, kimchi, and cabbage are all fermented foods that are high in probiotics, which help the body make GABA.

The B vitamins are GABA, which is made with the help of vitamins B6 and B12. Eat a lot of leafy veggies, whole grains, and legumes.

Tuning Down the Excitement of Glutamate

Cutting back on processed foods and simple sugars can help keep glutamate levels in check. Magnesium is a natural tranquilizer that helps keep the stimulating effects of glutamate in check. In your meals, eat bananas, nuts, seeds, and leafy greens.

A complete guide to maintaining healthy neurotransmitters called "Beyond the Plate."

Diet is a very important part of making neurotransmitters. Regular exercise makes your body produce chemicals that make you feel good, like endorphins and serotonin. Getting enough sleep is important for keeping neurotransmitters in check. Aim to get at least 7-8 hours of good sleep every night. Long-term worry can lower the amount; of neurotransmitters in the brain. Do things that help you relax, like yoga, meditation, or deep breathing.

You can take an active role in your own health by learning about the link between food and hormones. By living a healthy life and eating a balanced diet full of nutrients that improve your mood, you can make your brain work like a symphony, improving your happiness, focus, and general mental health.

Food as Brain Fuel

"Discover strategies to enhance your cognitive function and mental clarity through dietary choices."

Have you ever felt like your mind was cloudy? Everyone has times when they can't concentrate or remember things. What if, though, you could improve your brain power and mental sharpness by changing the way you eat? Good news: you can! Like an engine, your brain needs the right kind of fuel to work at its best. Food is like fuel for your brain. If you want to improve your brain power and mental focus through food choices, here are some ideas:

Pick Nutrients That Help Your Brain

Fat fish-like salmon, tuna, and sardines are great for your brain because they have these superfoods. They help you remember things, learn new things, and concentrate. Fish that is high in fat should be eaten at least twice a week. B vitamins, such as B6, B12, and folate, are important for brain health and are needed to turn food into energy. Eat a lot of nuts, whole grains, legumes, and leafy veggies. This vitamin helps you remember things and learn new things. Choline can be found in eggs, liver, and some nuts. These powerful things fight free radicals and keep brain cells from getting hurt. Veggies and fruits like bell peppers and leafy greens should be a part of your diet. Too much saturated and trans fats are bad for you, but good fats like those in nuts, avocados, and olive oil are important for brain health.

Getting Ready to Focus

A healthy breakfast gets your brain ready for the day. Choose foods that are high in whole grains, like oatmeal or whole-wheat toast with cream cheese and fruit. Brain fog and poor cognitive function can happen when you are dehydrated. Aim to drink eight glasses of water every day, but make changes based on how active you are. If you want to stay focused, don't eat sugary snacks because they can cause your blood sugar to drop. Choose snacks that are good for your brain, like yogurt with berries, nuts, or veggies with nut butter. Planning your meals and snacks ahead of time will help you make healthy choices throughout the day and keep you from snacking on bad things when you don't need to.

Beyond the Plate: Maxing Out Brainpower

Even though what you eat is very important. Regular exercise brings more blood to the brain, which helps new brain cells grow and strengthens brain function. Your brain fixes itself and puts together memories while you sleep. Aim to get at least 7-8 hours of good sleep every night. Do things that keep your mind active, like games, reading, or learning a new language. To keep your brain sharp, do things that keep it active. Long-term worry can make it harder to think clearly. Do things that help you relax, like yoga, meditation, or deep breathing.

Don't forget that consistency is key! Making these changes to your daily routine will give your brain the nutrients it needs to work at its best. You might be surprised at how much better your memory, focus, and general mental clarity get. Instead of snacking on sugary foods and processed foods, switch to a brain-boosting diet that will help you think and learn as much as you can!

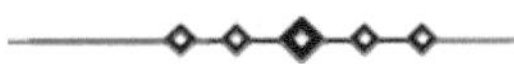

CHAPTER 10

Healing from the Inside Out

"Cellular Repair Through Nutrition"

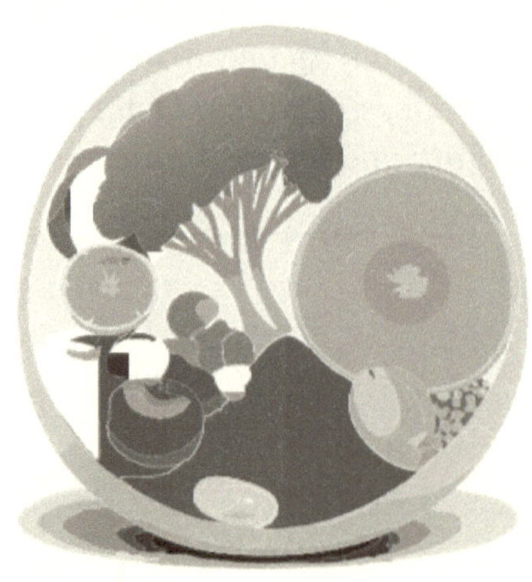

The Body's Repair Kit

"Understand how essential nutrients fuel cellular repair and wound healing."

The human body is a very strong machine that is always being worn down. Whether it's a small cut or a big surgery, our body's internal repair system heals the damage and gets things working again. But just like a car engine needs the right fuel to run well, our bodies need certain important nutrients to power this repair process, which is like having your repair kit inside you.

Getting to Know Cellular Repair

Think of your cells as millions of tiny construction workers who work nonstop to make and maintain your body. On their own, these cells die every day and need to be renewed. Also, cuts, scrapes, and even surgery can cause damage that needs to be fixed. To stop more damage, blood clotting systems are turned on. White blood cells rush to the hurt area to fight off infection and get rid of waste. To fix broken tissue, new cells are made. A protein called collagen helps close the wound and make it stronger by creating scar tissue.

Important Foods for the Repair Crew

In the same way, building workers need the right tools. Proteins are the building blocks of tissues and are required to make new cells and fix broken ones. Foods that are low in fat, like chicken, fish, beans, and lentils, provide amino acids that are needed to heal tissues. Vitamin C, a strong vitamin, helps the body make collagen, which is necessary for wounds to heal and scars to form. Vitamin C can be found in large amounts in bell peppers, broccoli, and citrus foods. Vitamin A is important for healthy skin and a strong immune system. It also helps cells grow and heal wounds. Vitamin A can be found in large amounts in sweet potatoes, carrots, and leafy greens. Zinc, this mineral, helps cells divide and the defense system work, which is both important for healing tissues. Zinc can be found in oysters, red meat, and pumpkin seeds. Staying hydrated is important for getting nutrients to all parts of the body, including the ones that are needed for repair. This is about omega-3 fatty acids. These fats that reduce inflammation help the body heal and may even help reduce swelling at the accident site. Salmon, tuna, and flaxseeds are all good sources of omega-3s.

Going Beyond the Plate: Improving Healing

A healthy, well-balanced diet full of these important nutrients is very important. Give your body the rest and sleep it needs to focus on healing. Keeping the skin clean and taking care of it the right way stops infections. Some health problems can make it harder to heal. For the best repair, it's important to take care of any underlying conditions like diabetes or long-term sicknesses.

It takes time to heal. By eating a healthy diet and taking care of wounds the right way, you can give your body the nutrients it needs to heal itself. If you are worried about how quickly a wound is healing or if it takes longer than expected to recover, talk to your doctor for specific help.

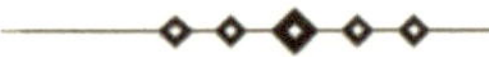

Building Blocks of Life

*"Explore the vital role of protein, antioxidants,
and specific vitamins and minerals in tissue
repair."*

Our bodies are like complicated fabrics made of trillions of tiny cells. These cells are always getting damaged, so they need to be fixed very carefully. Our bodies heal themselves in a symphony, using vital nutrients as the building blocks of life. This happens for everything from a small cut to major surgery. This piece talks about how important protein, antioxidants, and certain vitamins and minerals are for tissue repair and how they help keep the body healthy and strong.

The Cellular Symphony of Repair

Think of your body as a busy building site. Your cells, which are very small workers, are always renewing themselves. Cells that are damaged are broken down and reused, and new cells are carefully made. When you get hurt, like with cuts, scrapes, or surgery, you create more "construction zones" that need to be fixed. The most important thing is to stop the bleeding and keep the wound from getting worse. Platelets are a type of specialized blood cell that gather at the site of the wound and make a clot to close it up. Calling in the Troops": White blood cells, which are the body's defense system, rush to the hurt area. They keep infections away and get rid of the waste that damaged cells leave behind. This first swelling is important for healing, but it should go away on its own soon. Specialized cells called fibroblasts are triggered to make new collagen fibers. Collagen fibers are made of proteins and help tissues stay together. Depending on the type of damaged tissue, other specialized cells may also be called in to help make new healthy tissue. Scar Formation (Wound Healing) Collagen fibers are put down to make scar tissue as the wound heals. This scar tissue fills in the space and makes the hurt area strong again.

Protein: The Building Block for Repair

Protein is an important building block for cells. This molecule is made up of amino acids, which are the building blocks of cells. The body breaks down proteins during tissue repair and uses the amino acids to make new cells, fix broken cells, and make collagen. Getting enough protein is very important for healing.

The amino acids our bodies need can't be made by themselves. The nine important amino acids we need come from the food we eat. Chicken, fish, eggs, beans, and lentils are all lean protein foods that provide a full range of amino acids that help the body heal. Building new cells is like putting together Lego blocks out of amino acids. Protein synthesis is the main thing the body does to replace broken cells and make new ones for healthy tissue growth while tissue is being repaired. Certain amino acids are very important for collagen to be made. Collagen is the structure protein that gives new tissue strength and support. Proline, glycine, and hydroxyproline are some of the building blocks that collagen needs to work.

Protecting the Repair Crew with Antioxidants

Free radicals, which are molecules that are not solid, are made during the repair process. These free radicals can hurt cells and make it harder for them to heal. In the body's repair crew, antioxidants protect good cells from damage by getting rid of free radicals. Antioxidants can help lower inflammation, which is a normal part of healing but can get out of hand and make it harder to heal. Antioxidants get rid of free radicals, which stops them from hurting healthy cells and tissues around the damage. This helps the body recover more quickly and effectively. Some antioxidants, like those in berries, can make the blood flow better to the hurt area, making it easier for the body to get the oxygen and nutrients it needs to heal.

"The Essential Toolbox for Vitamins and Minerals"

Protein, antioxidants, and certain vitamins and minerals are also very important for tissue healing. This is vitamin C. This strong antioxidant is necessary for making collagen. It makes blood arteries stronger and boosts the immune system, which are both very important for healing. Vitamin C can be found in large amounts in bell peppers, broccoli, and citrus foods. This is vitamin A. Vitamin A is important for healthy skin and a strong immune system. It also helps cells grow and heal wounds. Vitamin A can be found in large amounts in sweet potatoes, carrots, and leafy greens. Zinc: This mineral helps cells divide and the defense system work, which are both very important for healing tissues. Zinc can be found in oysters, red meat, and pumpkin seeds. Not getting enough zinc can make it harder to heal. Vitamin D, This vitamin helps control how much calcium your body absorbs, which is important for bone health and repair. You can get a lot of vitamin D from fatty fish, eggs, and milk that has been supplemented. A number of B vitamins, especially B complex, help cells use energy and make new cells.

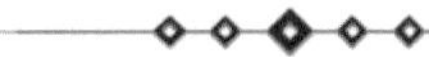

Optimizing Your Plate for Cellular Rejuvenation

"Learn strategies to create a dietary plan that promotes optimal cellular health."

Our bodies are complex environments made up of trillions of cells, which are the building blocks of life. Cellular health is very important for general health. Just like a well-kept yard grows well with the right care, our cells grow well when we eat smartly. In this guide, there are ways to make a food plan that supports good cell health, which will help you become healthy and strong.

Accept a Rainbow on Your Plate

Phytonutrients are plant-based chemicals that protect cells in nature. You can find them in fruits and veggies. They're like little guards that protect your cells from harm. There are many different phytonutrients in fruits and veggies, and each one is good for you in its own way. Every day, try to eat a wide range of colorful foods. Phytonutrients are mostly found in dark, leafy greens and foods with deep colors, like berries. Antioxidants are molecules that fight free radicals, and fruits and veggies are full of them. Free radicals are molecules that are not steady and can hurt cells and speed up the aging process. Antioxidants get rid of these free radicals, which is good for cell health and may lower the risk of getting chronic illnesses.

Put protein first for cellular renewal.

Building Blocks for Fix: As we've already talked about, proteins are what cells use to fix and renew themselves. It gives your body the necessary amino acids it needs to build and keep tissues healthy. Chicken, fish, beans, lentils, eggs, and low-fat yogurt are all good sources of lean protein that you can eat throughout the day.

Healthy Fats for Cellular Work

Fueling Cellular Processes: Too much saturated and trans fats are bad for you, but good fats like those in olive oil, nuts, seeds, avocados, and avocados are needed for cells to work. These fats are very important for carrying signals between cells, keeping membranes strong, absorbing nutrients when you can, and choosing healthy fats over harmful fats.

Water is the lifeblood of cells.

Important for Cellular Processes: Water is necessary for all body functions, including the health of cells. Water brings nutrients to cells, flushes out waste, and keeps the body's temperature stable. Dehydration can make cells less effective and mending processes more difficult. Aim to drink eight glasses of water every day, but make changes based on how active you are.

Ways to eat to help cells renew themselves

Cut down on processed foods. These foods usually have a lot of extra sugar, fats that are bad for you, and salt. These things can make inflammation and reactive stress worse, which are both bad for the health of cells. Limit the amount; of processed foods you eat and choose whole, raw foods whenever you can. Eating too much sugar can cause long-term inflammation and make it harder for cells to heal. Watch out for sugars that are hidden in processed foods and drinks. Instead of sweet treats, choose naturally sweet veggies. Take your time and enjoy your food. This helps your body process food and absorb nutrients better, which is good for your cells. The Mediterranean diet or the DASH diet, which is high in fruits, veggies, whole grains, and lean protein, may be good for your health and cells. Nonetheless, talk to a doctor or trained dietitian to find the eating plan that works best for your specific needs.

Going Beyond the Plate: A Whole-Pose Approach to Cellular Health

Doing regular physical exercise increases blood flow, which brings oxygen and nutrients to cells. Also, it helps get rid of trash and speeds up the repair of cells. Your body repairs and renews cells at the cellular level while you sleep. Aim to get at least 7-8 hours of good sleep every night. Long-term worry can hurt the health of cells. To improve the health of your cells, try stress-relieving activities like yoga, meditation, or deep breathing. Smoking and drinking too much booze can hurt cells and speed up the aging process.

Always do the same thing! You can build a foundation for optimal cellular health by making these changes to your food and way of life. You will be stronger and healthier if your cellular environment is healthy. Eat a variety of colors, focus on protein, stay hydrated, and live a healthy life. These are all important things to do to help your cells renew and your body's natural ability to grow.

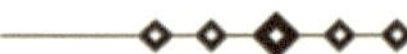

CHAPTER 11

Plant-Powered Recovery

"Exploring Plant-Based Diets"

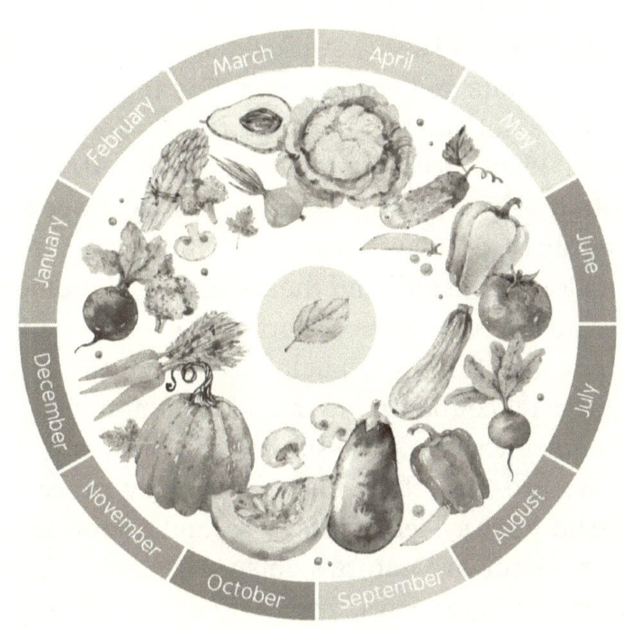

Harnessing the Power of Plants

"Discover the potential benefits of plant-based diets for promoting healing and overall well-being."

Plant-based diets have been popular in many countries around the world for hundreds of years because they believe they can help people stay healthy and live longer. In the past few years, scientific studies have started to show that eating mostly plants has a strong link to better health, healing, and avoiding disease. This piece goes into detail about how plant-based diets might help people heal and lay the groundwork for a long and healthy life.

There are many healthy foods on your plate.

Plant-based diets focus on whole plant foods like fruits, veggies, whole grains, legumes, nuts, and seeds. Antioxidants are molecules that fight free radicals, and fruits and veggies are full of them. Free radicals are molecules that are not stable and can hurt cells and make long-term illnesses worse. Plant-based diets contain many different kinds of antioxidants that help cells stay healthy and may lower the chance of getting chronic diseases. Plant-based foods have a lot of fiber, which is good for your stomach health and the balance of microbiomes in your gut. A healthy gut microbiome is important for your general health and immune system, and it may even help your body heal. Fruits, veggies, and whole grains all contain many important vitamins and minerals, such as folate, magnesium, potassium, and vitamins A, C, E, and K. These nutrients are important for many bodily processes, such as protecting the immune system, fixing cells, and healing wounds. These chemicals from plants are nature's defense system and may be good for your health in several ways. The anti-inflammatory properties of some phytonutrients can help the body heal and lower the risk of chronic illnesses.

Plant-Based Health Benefits for Healing

Some plant-based foods, like whole grains, fruits, and veggies, naturally reduce inflammation. Several health problems are linked to chronic inflammation. A plant-based diet may help lower inflammation, which may speed up healing and possibly decrease the risk of getting chronic illnesses. Plant-based foods tend to have less cholesterol and saturated fat, which can make the blood flow better. Enough blood flow is important for getting oxygen and nutrients to all parts of the body's cells, which helps the healing process. Plant-based meals tend to have fewer calories per serving and more fiber, which makes you feel full and may help you control your weight. Keeping a healthy weight can be good for your health in general and may help you heal after surgery or an accident. A well-balanced plant-based diet is full of whole grains, fruits, and veggies gives your immune system the nutrients it needs to stay healthy. A strong immune system is important for preventing infections and speeding up the mending process.

Besides Healing the Body

Studies show a link between eating mostly plants and having better happiness and brain function. The gut bacteria are affected by what you eat, and this can affect your mental health. Plant-based diets may have a positive effect on gut bacteria, which could be good for mental health. People who eat mostly plants have a lower chance of getting many long-term diseases, like heart disease, type 2 diabetes, and some cancers. These long-term problems can make it harder to heal and be healthy in general. A plant-based diet might help keep you fit and keep you from getting sick.

Choosing to live a plant-based life

You don't have to go all-in or all-out when switching to a plant-based diet. "Start Small" means to start by eating more plant-based meals every day. You can start by eating only one or two plant-based meals a day and add more as you feel ready. Plant-based options like tofu, lentils, legumes, and tofu are tasty and high in protein. Look through ideas to find new ways to make your meals more interesting by adding plant-based protein sources. Whole, raw plant foods should be chosen over packaged or processed foods. This will help you get the most out of the fiber and important nutrients that plants offer. A registered dietitian can help you make a plant-based meal plan that is healthy and fits your wants and tastes.

Don't forget that consistency is key! You can use the healing power of plants to improve your general health and well-being by slowly adding more plant-based meals to your daily routine and expanding your plant-based food choices.

Fueling Your Body with Plant-Based Protein

"Learn about complete and incomplete proteins and strategies for getting enough protein on a plant-based diet."

Protein is the building block of life and is very important for many bodily processes, such as keeping the immune system healthy and building and repairing tissues. Animal goods, such as meat, poultry, and dairy, have long been thought to be the best source of protein. But more and more people are choosing plant-based diets, which makes me wonder: Is it possible to get enough protein on a plant-based diet? There is no doubt that the answer is yes! There are many types of protein in plants, and if you plan ahead, you can make sure your body gets all the protein it needs to stay healthy.

Complete and incomplete proteins: what you need to know

Amino acids, which are the building blocks of cells, make up proteins. Of the 20 amino acids that are out there, our bodies can make 11 of them. The other nine, though, are called vital amino acids, and we need to get them from food. All nine necessary amino acids are found in these protein sources in the right amounts for the body. Complete proteins can be found in foods like meat, chicken, fish, eggs, and dairy. One or more of the necessary amino acids are missing from these protein sources. You can make a "complementary protein" that gives your body all the amino acids it needs, though, by smartly mixing different plant-based protein sources throughout the day.

Powerhouse of Plant-Based Protein

There are many protein-rich plants to choose from. Peas, beans, lentils, and chickpeas are all great sources of fiber and protein. About 18 grams of protein can be found in one cup of cooked beans! You can try different kinds and add them to salads, soups, stews, or sauces.

Tofu, tempeh, and edamame are all made from soybeans and are good sources of all nine essential amino acids. These are versatile foods that go well in a lot of different meals, from scrambled eggs and stir-fries to marinades and sauces. Peanuts, walnuts, cashews, chia seeds, and hemp seeds are just a few of the nuts and seeds that are high in protein, good fats, and fiber. You can eat them as a snack, put them on yogurt or salads, or spread nut butter into sandwiches. Whole grains like quinoa, oats and brown rice help you meet your daily protein needs, but they aren't as protein-dense as some other foods. You can eat quinoa as a side dish or add it to salads and bowls because it is a full protein source.

How to Get the Most Out of Plant-Based Protein

You don't have to cut back on energy when you switch to a plant-based diet. A variety of plant-based protein sources should be eaten throughout the day. Making sure you get all the amino acids your body needs is important. When you pair up incomplete plant-based proteins, you can make proteins that work well together and provide all nine necessary amino acids. You could put peanut butter on whole-wheat bread, beans, and rice, or whole-wheat tacos and black beans. Make sure you include enough protein sources in your meals and snacks by planning them ahead of time. Look into plant-based recipes to get new ideas for how to add protein to your food. Although not high in protein, leafy greens like spinach and kale do contain some protein and are important for your health. Plant-based protein shakes made from pea protein, brown rice protein, or hemp protein can be helpful for people who need more protein or are having trouble getting enough protein from food alone.

Quality Matters More Than Quantity of Protein

It's important to make sure you get enough protein, but the quality of the protein is also important. Some animal protein sources are high in fatty fat and cholesterol, but plant-based protein sources are often high in fiber, healthy fats, vitamins, and minerals, as well as protein. Because of this, plant-based protein is a healthy pick that is high in nutrients.

Join the journey towards plant-based protein.

Fueling your body with plant-based energy can be fun and satisfying. You can make sure your body gets all the protein it needs to grow by trying out different plant-based protein sources, planning your meals, and mixing them in smart ways. Always being the same is important! Over time, add more plant-based protein choices to your diet. You will be amazed at how plants can heal and fuel your body.

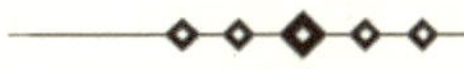

Plant-Based Abundance

"Explore the diverse and delicious world of plant-based foods to create satisfying and nourishing meals."

Plant-based food is like a colorful fabric with lots of different tastes, textures, and colors. An entirely plant-based diet does not limit your food choices; instead, it opens up a world of delicious and healthy food options. This piece talks about the wide range of tasty plant-based foods that are available. It will help you make meals that are both tasty and good for you.

Welcome the Rainbow to Your Plate

There are so many delicious fruits and veggies in nature, and each one has its special flavor and set of nutrients. From the bright sweetness of berries and melons to the earthy richness of roasted root veggies and the crispness of leafy greens, discover the wide range of tastes found in plants. Fruits and veggies are full of vitamins, minerals, antioxidants, and fiber, all of which are very good for your health and well-being.

Grains for Strength and Longevity

Whole grains are a filling base for your meals. They contain complex carbohydrates that give you long-lasting energy and dietary fiber that keeps your gut healthy. Quinoa, amaranth, and teff are all types of ancient grains that are high in fiber and protein. You can eat them in bowls with meat, pilafs, or even mush. Find out how grains from around the world can be used in many ways. A lot of Asian food is made with brown rice, and couscous gives salads and stews a great structure.

The History of Legume

The food group legumes, which includes beans, lentils, and chickpeas, is very healthy. When mixed with grains, they make a full vegetarian protein source because they are high in protein, fiber, and important vitamins and minerals. Legumes are used in a wide range of dishes around the world, from Indian dals and Moroccan tagines to Mexican black bean soup and Italian pasta e fagioli. You can eat legumes in burgers, soups, stews, salads, dips, and even sauces. Try different combinations of herbs and spices to make a flavor explosion.

Nuts and seeds are like little power plants in nature.

Nuts and seeds have a lot of fiber, vitamins, minerals, good fats, and protein. Nuts and seeds are a great healthy snack to take with you. You can eat them raw, roast them, or make nut kinds of butter out of them. Add nuts and seeds to salads, stir-fries, curries, and even sweets to make them more-interesting and healthy.

Alternatives to milk made from plants

Almond milk, soy milk, oat milk, and coconut milk all have different tastes and textures that make them great for breakfast, smoothies, coffee, or just drinking on their own. You can bake with plant-based kinds of milk, make creamy sauces, or make tasty vegan yogurt replacements.

The Symphony of Spices

Herbs and spices are the unsung stars of plant-based cooking. Explore the world of spices, from the spicy flavors of Indian stews to the sweet and smoky notes of paprika and the tangy lemongrass. Herbs and spices that are fresh and those that are dried have different tastes. Dried spices pack a stronger flavor punch, while fresh herbs add a splash of color to your food.

Beyond the Plate: Making Plans and Getting Ready

It's not hard to make plant-based meals that taste great and fill you up. Take some time to make a plan for the week's meals. This makes sure you have all the items you need and keeps you from making unhealthy choices at the last minute. There are a lot of tasty and interesting plant-based recipes on the internet and in cookbooks.

Try out different tastes and types of food. Make sure you have whole grains, beans, nuts, seeds, canned veggies, and plant-based milks in your pantry at all times. This makes it easy to make healthy food. Try something new! Do not be afraid to try new tastes and textures. When it comes to plant-based nutrition, the options are endless.

CHAPTER 12

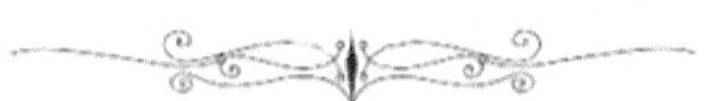

Unveiling Hidden Sensitivities

"The Strategic Approach to Elimination Diets"

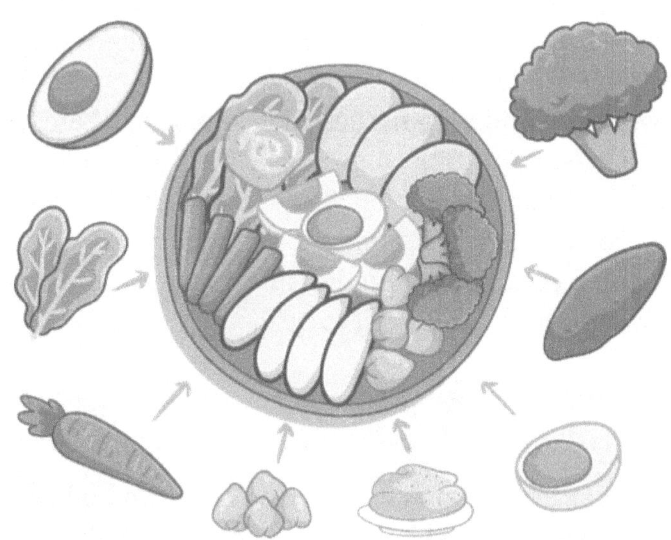

Identifying Food Sensitivities

"Understand how food sensitivities can impact your recovery and explore methods for identifying them."

Food sensitivities, which are not the same as food allergies, can make it harder for you to get better after an illness, surgery, or accident. Food sensitivities are not as bad as food allergies, which cause a strong immune response. However, they can still cause problems that last for a long time and make it harder to heal and be healthy generally. Food sensitivities may affect recovery, and this piece talks about how to find out if you have one so you can make the most of your healing journey.

Food Sensitivities and Recovery is the title of the book.

Food allergies can show up in many ways, often with mild but long-lasting symptoms that can make it harder to get better. Food allergies can cause low-level inflammation, which makes it harder for the body to heal itself naturally. Inflammation can make wounds hurt more, take longer to heal, and stop tissues from repairing themselves. Food sensitivities can lead to stomach problems like gas, bloating, diarrhea, or not being able to go to the toilet. These can make it harder to absorb nutrients, which is important for healing. Food allergies can make you tired, make you feel exhausted all the time, and give you muscle aches, which lowers the energy you need to heal.

Finding the Root Cause: Recognizing Food Allergies

Finding out what foods someone is sensitive to can be like a mystery. This is an organized method in which you cut out foods that you think might be a trigger for a set amount of time (usually two to four weeks) and then slowly add them back in one by one. If the symptoms change after return, this could be a sign of sensitivity. If you want to try this method, you should talk to a doctor or trained dietitian first. It can be helpful to keep a thorough food journal for a few weeks. Write down everything you eat and drink and any signs you have. This can help find patterns and possible causes. Some doctors may suggest an IgG blood test to find out if someone might be sensitive to certain foods, but the results aren't always clear-cut. Some people disagree with these tests, though, and their accuracy is called into question. It's important to talk to your doctor about the limits of this test before you decide to get it. It's important to speak to a doctor or certified dietitian before starting an elimination diet or figuring out what test results mean. They can walk you through the process and make sure it is safe and effective for finding out if you are sensitive to certain foods.

Improving Your Road to Recovery

Once you know what foods set off your symptoms, you should either not eat them at all or eat very little of them. This lets your body heal without having to deal with sensitivity reactions. Choose whole foods that are high in nutrients, like fruits, veggies, whole grains, and lean protein sources. This makes sure that your body gets the building blocks it needs to heal. A registered dietitian can help you create a personalized plan that takes into account your food allergies and gives you the nutrients you need to heal at your best.

The Way Back to Health

Finding out about and taking care of food sensitivities can make a huge difference in your healing. By finding the secret causes and putting a healthy diet first, you can speed up your body's natural healing processes and make a full recovery possible. Always being the same is important. You can set yourself up for long-term health and repair by sticking to a personalized plan and being aware of any possible sensitivities.

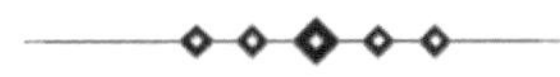

The Power of Elimination

"Learn the principles of elimination diets and how to utilize them effectively."

Our bodies are complex environments, and the foods we eat can sometimes cause reactions we don't want. These responses, which are sometimes called food sensitivities, can show up in different ways and hurt our health and well-being. It can be hard to figure out what is causing these issues. The elimination diet is a strong way to find the foods that are hurting your health without you even knowing it. This piece goes into detail about the ideas behind elimination diets, looks at how well they work, and gives you the information you need to use them correctly.

How to Understand Food Sensitivities

Food allergies and food sensitivities are not the same thing. Food allergies cause a strong immune reaction, which leads to immediate symptoms that could be life-threatening, such as anaphylaxis. On the other hand, people with food sensitivities have a less severe reaction that is controlled by their immune system or gut system. Symptoms can be mild and appear later than expected, which makes it hard to diagnose. Skin problems like eczema or acne or headaches Joint pain or muscle aches Feeling tired and unmotivated

A Detective's Approach to the Elimination Diet

A structured method called an elimination diet is used to find foods that make your body react badly. Like a spy game, you gradually get rid of foods that you think might be causing your symptoms and watch to see if your symptoms change. In this step, you have to stop eating a certain group of foods that usually cause problems for a set amount of time, two to four weeks. Dairy, gluten, eggs, soy, nuts, legumes, maize, and some fruits and veggies may be on this list. A registered dietitian or health care worker can help you make a personalized list of things to avoid based on what you think are your triggers. Observation During the elimination phase, keep a food log and write down everything you eat and drink. Also, write down any signs you have, including how bad they are and when they happen. Keeping such thorough records is im-important for finding patterns and possible triggers. You'll start the return phase after the elimination phase is over. Here, you'll slowly add back in the foods you cut out, usually taking a few days between each one. This gives your body time to respond and figure out what might set it off. Keep writing down what you eat and how you feel in your food log during reintroduction. You can make changes to your food based on what you saw during the reintroduction phase. If a certain food makes you sick, you may decide to stop eating it or limit how much you eat of it.

How to Get the Most Out of Your Elimination Diet

Following an elimination diet is possible on your own, but it can be very helpful to talk to a doctor or trained dietitian first. They can help you make a personalized list of foods to avoid, make sure you get enough nutrition during the process, and read your food log to find possible triggers. Put whole, raw foods at the top of your list during the elimination phase. This makes sure you get the nutrients you need while lowering the chance of eating processed foods that contain secret triggers. For an elimination plan to work, you must carefully record what you eat in a journal. It's important to keep accurate records of what you eat and drink, as well as any symptoms you have, to find trends and possible triggers. It is very important to follow the elimination and reintroduction stages. If you skip steps or add foods too fast, it can be hard to figure out what's wrong. Finding out what foods make you sensitive can take some time. It might take a few weeks to finish an elimination diet, and you might not see effects right away. For best results, be patient and steady.

Pros and cons of elimination diets

Doing away with a lot of foods at once can make it hard to find the exact cause. You can stop eating food that wasn't bothering you and then later add back a real trigger. Cutting out a lot of food groups

can make you more likely not to get enough of some nutrients,
especially if you don't plan your diet well. Talking to a doctor or
certified dietitian can help you make sure you're getting all the
nutrients you need during the process. Elimination diets can be hard
to stick to because they are so restricted. They might not be right for
everyone, especially people who don't have a lot of means or who
already have health problems.

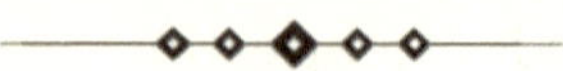

Reintroduction Roadmap

"Discover strategies for safely reintroducing eliminated foods and creating a long-term sustainable plan."

You've found the foods that might be hurting your health after the hard work of the elimination diet. Now comes the most important part: return. During this step, you slowly start eating the foods you had to give up, watching your body's reaction, and then making a personalized, long-term diet plan. This piece gives you safe and effective ways to reintroduce food, which can lead to a healthy and happy relationship with food.

The Fine Art of Reintroduction:

The dance of reintroduction is one of exploring and observing. You will slowly add back the foods you stopped eating, one at a time while paying close attention to how your body reacts. Make a plan for how you will do the reintroduction before you start. Choose the order in which you will reintroduce foods. Usually, it would help if you started with the ones you don't think will cause an issue. Look over any notes or advice that your doctor or trained dietitian has given you. It's important to be patient. Reintroduce each food one at a time, giving three to five days between each one. This gives your body plenty of time to adapt, which makes it easier to figure out what went wrong if something bad does happen. For each reintroduction, eat a modest amount of the food that was removed, preferably without eating anything else. This "challenge dose" helps to make any possible response stronger, which makes it easier to spot. During reintroduction, keep your very detailed food log. Please write down the name of the food you reintroduced, how much you ate, and any symptoms you have, along with how bad they are and when they happen. Keeping such thorough records is important for finding patterns and possible triggers.

How to Find the Criminals

Watch how your body reacts to each food as you reintroduce it. When you eat certain foods and then have bloating, gas, diarrhea, or constipation, these can be signs that something is wrong. If acne, eczema, or other skin problems show up after return, this could mean that the person is sensitive. If you get headaches or migraines again after eating a certain food, it could be a cause. If joint pain or muscle aches come back after return it could mean that the body is sensitive. If you feel tired or have low energy after eating a certain food, that could be a sign.

Putting together your food map

You can make a personalized food map based on what you saw during your return to help you make food choices in the future. Foods that consistently make your symptoms worse should probably be taken out of your diet or eaten much less often in the future. If some foods make your responses mild or only sometimes happen, you might want to limit how much of them you eat and rotate them in your diet. As long as you don't have any bad responses to the foods listed below, you can eat them as part of a healthy plan.

Making a Plan That Will Last

The end goal is not just to find triggers but also to make a healthy eating plan that is enjoyable and easy to stick to. A diet full of whole, unprocessed foods like fruits, veggies, whole grains, and lean protein sources should be your top priority. This makes sure you get a lot of different nutrients that your body needs. Finding new tasty foods that you can still eat can make sticking to a limited diet more fun. Look into other types of food and ideas that fit your needs. When you eat, pay attention to your body's signals for when you're hungry or full. Enjoy your food, and don't do anything else while you're eating. Having a network of people who can help you along the way can be very helpful, whether it's a registered dietitian, a healthcare worker, a friend, or a family member. See the changes you're making to your food as a way to improve your health, not as a punishment. Enjoy the things you've done well, and try to feel your best.

Don't forget that there is no one-size-fits-all solution. It's important to make sure that your diet plan fits your specific goals and is safe for you. There may be setbacks along the way, and reintroduction may not always go in a straight line. Keep listening to your body and being kind to yourself. You can build a healthy, long-lasting relationship with food that supports your health and well-being if you work at it and look at it as a whole.

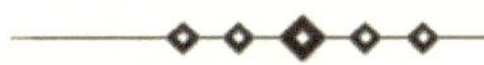

CHAPTER 13

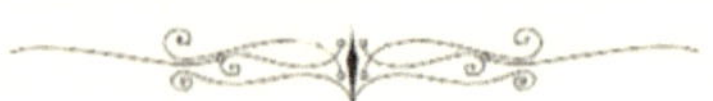

Transformations Through Food

"Stories of Renewal"

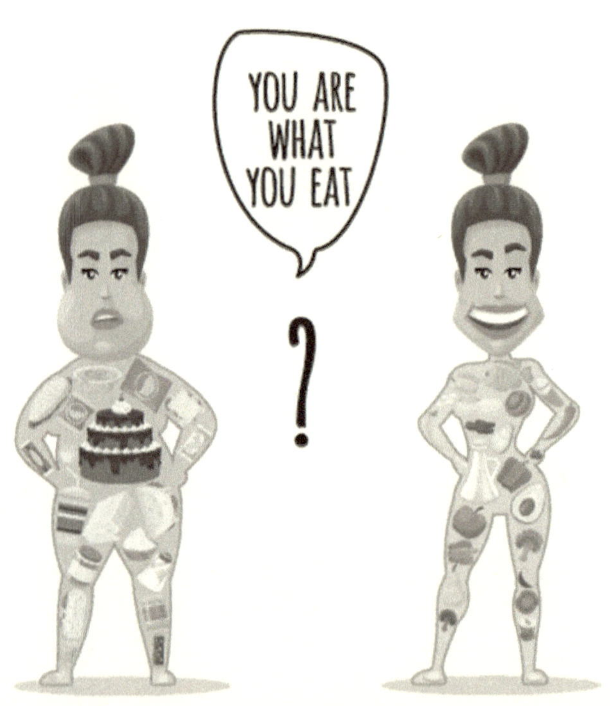

The Power of Inspiration

"Dive into inspiring stories of individuals who used nutrition to heal and reclaim their health."

Food is more than just sustenance – it's a powerful tool for healing and transformation. Countless individuals have harnessed the power of nutrition to overcome health challenges and reclaim their vitality. These inspiring stories serve as a testament to the profound impact that mindful eating can have on our well-being.

From Chronic Fatigue to Ironman: Sarah's Story

Sarah, once plagued by chronic fatigue and digestive issues, resigned herself to a life of low energy and discomfort. However, a chance encounter with a registered dietitian sparked a change. By adopting a whole-food, plant-based diet, Sarah experienced a remarkable transformation. Her fatigue subsided, digestive issues vanished, and she discovered a newfound energy she never knew possible. Inspired by her improved health, Sarah embarked on a journey to complete an Ironman triathlon, a feat she once thought unimaginable.

Sugar Detox and a Life Transformed: Michael's Journey

Michael, a self-proclaimed sugar addict, battled weight gain, lethargy, and constant cravings. After a health scare forced him to confront his dietary habits, Michael embarked on a sugar detox. The initial withdrawal was challenging, but as the detox progressed, he noticed a dramatic shift. He lost weight effortlessly, his energy levels soared, and his chronic headaches disappeared. This newfound health fueled a passion for fitness, and Michael became a personal trainer, inspiring others to reclaim their health through mindful eating.

Healing Autoimmunity with Food: The Tale of Olivia

Olivia was diagnosed with a debilitating autoimmune disease, leaving her feeling hopeless and overwhelmed. Traditional treatment offered limited relief, but Olivia refused to give up. She embarked on a research journey, discovering the powerful connection between food and autoimmunity. By eliminating inflammatory foods and adopting a gut-healing diet, Olivia experienced a dramatic turnaround. Her symptoms lessened, her energy returned, and she finally found a path to manage her condition. Olivia now uses her experience to empower others with autoimmune diseases, demonstrating the power of food as medicine.

Beyond Weight Loss: John's Transformation

John's journey with nutrition wasn't solely about weight loss. He grappled with chronic pain and a feeling of overall sluggishness. By incorporating anti-inflammatory foods and learning about portion control, John started noticing changes beyond the scale. His pain subsided, his sleep improved, and he felt a renewed sense of vitality. This experience fueled a passion for healthy cooking, and John now uses his story to inspire others to focus on whole-body wellness through mindful food choices.

These are just a few stories among countless others. Every individual's journey with nutrition is unique. The common thread is the transformative power of food. By approaching nutrition with intention and knowledge, we unlock the potential to heal our bodies, reclaim our health, and live with renewed vitality.

Inspired to start your own journey?

- ✓ Consult a registered dietitian for personalized guidance.

- ✓ Explore cookbooks and websites dedicated to healthy eating.

- ✓ Connect with online communities focused on nutrition and wellness.

A healthy relationship with food is a lifelong journey. Embrace the power of inspiration, celebrate the success stories, and embark on your own path to vibrant health through mindful eating.

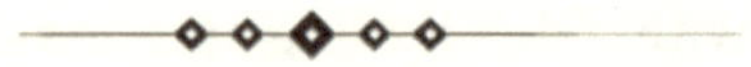

From Struggle to Strength

"Learn from real-life experiences of overcoming challenges and achieving transformation through food."

We get hit by curveballs in life. Problems like these can sometimes show up in our bodies, making us feel tired and lost. But even in the middle of the struggle, there is a strong way to change things: food. This piece talks about real-life examples of people who used nutrition to get through tough times and make amazing changes. They can help you find your way to a better, more vibrant life through their stories.

"Beating Crohn's: Emily's Story of Gut Healing"

Emily's fight with Crohn's disease, an inflammatory gut disease, was her whole life. She felt lost because she was in constant pain, had crippling flare-ups, and had to follow a strict diet. Traditional medicine didn't help much, and most people were told to eat plain, uninteresting foods. Emily, on the other hand, refused to accept the limits. After doing a lot of studies, she found that her condition was linked to gut health. She started an elimination diet with the help of a trained dietitian, carefully figuring out which foods set off her symptoms and avoiding them. Slowly, she began eating things that are good for your gut again, like fermented vegetables, bone broth, and prebiotics. It was amazing how things changed. She finally found a way to deal with her condition; her symptoms got better, and her flare-ups happened less often and with less pain. Emily's story shows how a personalized diet can help with gut health and managing chronic diseases.

David's Journey of Taking Back Control: From Food Addiction to Mindfulness

David's life was all about food. He always wanted food, ate too much, and felt guilty about it. He had a problem with food addiction, which is shamed and ignored by many. Using old ways like counting calories only gave short-term results. But a chance meeting with a mindful eating guide made them change. David learned to recognize the feelings that made him eat too much and used mindful eating methods to improve his relationship with food. He focused on intuitive eating, which means he paid attention to his body's signals for when it was hungry and full, and he enjoyed every bite. Over time, David's compulsive cravings went away, and he got back in charge of his food. Food was no longer a cause of shame; it became fuel. It's clear from David's story that mindfulness can help people beat food addiction and develop a healthy connection with food.

Beyond the Wheelchair: Sarah's Story of Living with Chronic Pain

Sarah had continuous pain that kept her in a wheelchair and controlled her life. Doctors prescribed medicines that helped with the symptoms but not the cause. Sarah was determined to find a solution, so she did a lot of studies on foods that reduce inflammation. She cut out foods that make her body hurt, like processed sugars and unhealthy fats, and started eating lots of fruits, veggies, omega-3 fatty acids, and whole grains. It wasn't easy, but the end result changed my life. Over time, the pain got better, her energy level rose, and she traded in her wheelchair for walking sticks. Sarah's story shows how anti-inflammatory foods can help people with chronic pain get their movement back.

The story of Michael's journey to love himself, from binge eating to body positivity.

Michael had a problem with binge eating, which was made worse by having a bad opinion of himself and always having to fight with the scale. Restrictive diets made the loop worse. But an online group for body-positive people changed their minds. Michael learned to focus on giving his body what it needs instead of putting limits on it. He looked for tasty, healthy meals and started eating more intuitively. His relationship with his body changed along with his relationship with food. The focus changed from weight to health in general. Self-love and body positivity are very important for breaking bad eating habits and building a healthy relationship with food, as Michael's story shows.

These are just a few stories that show how food can change things. Food isn't just fuel; it's a strong tool that can help us get through tough times, get our health back, and make amazing changes.

Are you feeling ready to start your own journey? Here are some ideas

They can help you make a plan that works for you and your specific needs and problems. For the best nutrition, focus on fruits, vegetables, whole grains, and lean protein sources. Learn to pay attention to your body's signals for hunger and fullness and develop a more mindful relationship with food. Be patient with yourself and celebrate your progress, no matter how small. Get in touch with a coach, therapist, or online community for support and encouragement.

Don't forget that change is a process, not a goal. You can find your own way to a healthier and more satisfying life by getting ideas from these true stories, learning about the power of food, and moving towards mindful eating.

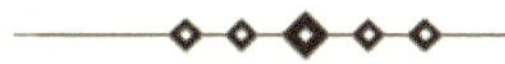

You Are Not Alone

"Find encouragement and connection through the shared journeys of others on the path to healing."

On the way to healing, you may feel alone at times. We deal with pain in our bodies, trouble in our emotions, and the crushing sense of being lost in a maze of unknowns. But in the middle of the battle, there is a strong source of comfort: hearing about other people's experiences. The stories of people who have been through the same thing before can be like beacons in the fog. They give you hope, validation, and a sense of belonging. Imagine that Sarah has a long-term sickness that makes her feel tired and hopeless. Traditional methods don't help much, and most people think you should follow a strict diet. Still, Sarah learns a lot by reading about the struggles of other people who have been through similar things. She knows how gut-healing foods can change her life, how important it is to figure out her triggers, and how her emotions are connected to food. At once, she's not by herself. With this new information and a sense of belonging, Sarah starts a personalized path to getting her health back. David's story hits home in a different way. He feels defeated and ashamed because he is stuck in the never-ending circle of food addiction. Counting calories only works for a short time, and fighting his cravings all the time wears him out. Then, he finds an online group that is all about thoughtful eating. Here, he meets people who understand how hard things are for him. He figures out what makes him feel bad, learns how to eat mindfully, and starts to have a better relationship with food. The shame begins to go away, and hope and friendship take its place. David realizes that he's not fighting this battle by himself. With the help of his new friends, he begins to take back charge. Michael's life is filled with pain that won't go away. Since he has to use a wheelchair, the constant pain takes away his freedom and joy. Some medicines doctors prescribe help with the symptoms, but they don't treat the cause. Michael looks into foods that reduce inflammation because he needs an answer badly. He finds a huge number of stories of people who got better by changing what they ate. Michael starts a journey to add anti-inflammatory foods to his diet after hearing about their experiences. It takes a long time, but the end result changes your life. He feels less pain, has more energy, and remembers how much fun it is to move. Michael's story shows how powerful it is to share what you know and how strong it is to be part of a group. These are just a few of the many stories that people on the way to healing have told. The power of link is what ties all of these stories together, even though they are all different. We find new opportunities, gain useful knowledge, and find the strength to keep going when we learn from others. We know that the problems we're having aren't impossible to solve and that there are people in our community who are here for us.

Sharing weakness is a huge source of strength. We make it possible for others to talk about their problems when we do. Support groups, online communities, and even casual chats can help people feel like they fit in and are understood. Sharing our stories not only makes us feel less alone, but it also encourages and helps other people on their own paths. Healing doesn't always happen in a straight line. Setbacks, times of doubt, and days when it doesn't look like the way forward are all part of life. Don't forget that you're not alone. You can get through the hard times and come out stronger, healthier, and more in control than ever before by drawing strength from the experiences of others, embracing the power of connection, and enjoying even the smallest wins. Your way to a better, healthier tomorrow can be lit by the light of other people's travels.

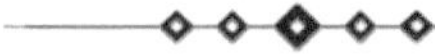

CHAPTER 14

The Healing Circle

"Leveraging the Power of Shared Support"

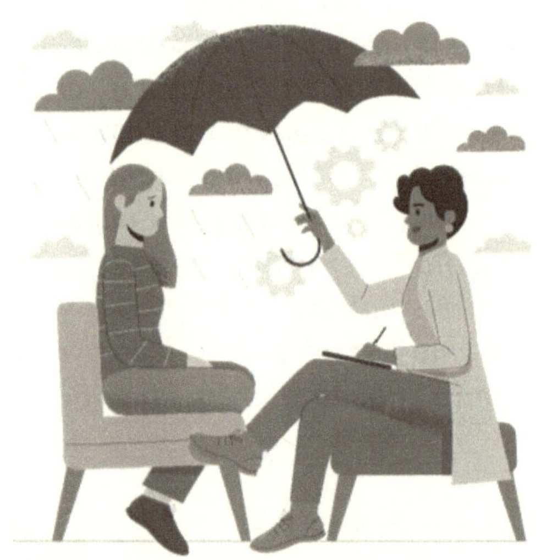

Building Your Support System

"Discover the importance of connecting with others on a similar healing journey."

To heal, you may need to be strong, take care of yourself, and stay motivated all the way through. But getting through this road doesn't have to be done by yourself. You can make a big difference in your healing process by putting together a strong support system of people who understand your problems and celebrate your successes.

Sharing a story can be very powerful.

Imagine that Sarah has a long-term illness that makes her feel alone and confused. Traditional methods don't help much, and most people think you should follow a strict diet. But Sarah finds a wealth of information by getting in touch with people who have been through the same thing. She learns how gut-healing foods can change her life, how important it is to figure out what foods set her off, and how food affects her emotions. At once, she's not by herself. With this new information and a sense of connection, Sarah starts a personalized path to regaining her health with the help of other people's experiences.

How to Find Your Tribe

There are different ways that the support system you build can look. You can find people who are going through the same health problems in online groups that are just for that topic. The safest place to share your stories, ask questions, and find comfort in being vulnerable is in a support group, whether it's in person or online. Talking to friends or family who have been through their own health problems can help you understand and feel better.

The Good Things About Being Connected

Having a good support system can help you in many ways. Talking about your problems with people who "get it" can make you feel a lot better. You'll feel better knowing you're not alone, and their understanding can help you feel less alone. Support services have a lot of useful information. Reading about how other people have dealt with similar problems can teach you brand new strategies, help you find tools, and give you useful information. Seeing other people heal can be exceptionally inspiring and motivating. Their stories can provide you with hope again and push you to keep going when things get hard. Having people who care about you can help you stick to your health goals. Telling other people about your challenges and success can help you stay on track and motivated.

Supporting each other by building bridges

Putting together a support system takes time and work. Think about what kind of help you need. Do you need someone to hold you responsible, listen, or give you advice?

Look for people who are going through the same problems in online communities, support groups, or through suggestions from healthcare professionals. It can be scary to talk about your problems, but it's the only way to build real relationships. It takes work on both ends to create a support system. Help other people get better by being there for them.

A strong support system is not a magic bullet, but it is a very helpful thing as you heal. You can build a network of strength and support by connecting with people who understand your struggles and celebrate your successes. This will help you take a more empowered and fulfilling road to health and well-being.

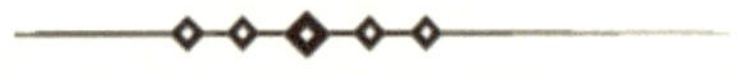

The Strength in Numbers

"Explore online communities, and support groups, or find a recovery buddy for encouragement and accountability."

It can be hard and lonely to get better, whether you're sick physically or emotionally. As we take steps into new areas, we often deal with loneliness, worry, and a constant "what if" feeling. But even with these problems, there is a strong tool that can help: there is strength in numbers. Connecting with people who are going through the same things as us opens up a world of support, encouragement, and responsibility that helps us move forward in our quest for health and happiness.

How powerful online communities can be

Think of Amelia was told she has a long-term inflammatory disease. The new symptoms and huge amount of knowledge make her feel lost and confused. However, after a quick search on the internet, Amelia found a lively online group that was just for people with her condition. Here, she meets people who have been through the same things she has and can relate. They talk about what they've been through, give each other useful help, and celebrate each other's wins. Amelia no longer feels alone all of a sudden. Amelia feels like she can take charge of her health now that she feels like she belongs and has learned a lot from the community's combined wisdom. A wide range of health issues are talked about in online groups. People who are dealing with chronic illnesses or food addictions can find safety in these online havens where they can meet, share their stories, and make friends. Online venues can be especially helpful for people who aren't sure how to talk about things in public because they are anonymous.

Pros Besides Connection

Message boards and online groups are great places to find a lot of useful information. You can find new ways to deal with problems, find different kinds of treatment, and get useful advice from more experienced people who have been through the same issues. Seeing other people's strengths and growth can be a powerful source of motivation. When things are going badly, reading about people who overcame huge problems can give you hope again. Online groups give you a safe place to talk about your worries, fears, and frustrations with people who understand. Knowing you're not alone can make you feel a lot better when you're feeling lonely and hopeless. There are moderators or even healthcare experts in many online communities who can help people, answer specific questions, and give them advice. Discovering the ideal online group can be a life-changing event. Keep an eye out for platforms that meet your unique needs and create a welcoming and supportive space. It would help if you weren't afraid to lurk and watch before you join in.

How Powerful In-Person Help Is

There are many good things about internet communities, but there's something special about meeting someone in person. Support groups give you a safe place to talk about your journey with people who understand how hard it is. Being able to connect with someone on a deeper level, show support without words, and make long friendships can be very empowering.

How to Find a Support Group

You can find support groups in your area at hospitals, clinics, community centers, or even online sites that list local groups. When picking a support group, think about things like its size, location, and main goal. If the first group you try doesn't work out, don't give up. It's important to find a group where you can feel safe and heard.

What's good about shared vulnerability

Meeting with a support group in person is a different way to get help. Telling a group about your goals and problems can make you feel responsible, which can keep you on track with your healing. Hearing that other people who have been through the same thing understand

and agree with you can be very comforting and help ease feelings of loneliness. Members of support groups can share useful ways to deal with problems, useful tools, and advice they've learned from their own experiences. The shared understanding and camaraderie in a support group can help people become friends for life, giving them support beyond the weekly meetings.

How to Find a Recovery Buddy

Sometimes, connecting with someone more personally is what you need. A healing buddy is someone you can talk to regularly who is going through the same thing you are. While you're alone, you can hold each other accountable, enjoy your wins, and share resources.

How to Find the Right Buddy

Find someone who is going through the same things you are and who you can trust and connect with. This person could be a family member, a friend, or someone you meet in an online community or support group.

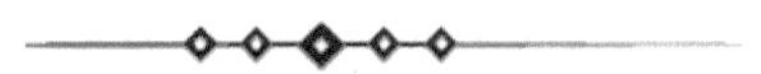

Giving Back and Paying it Forward

Going through the process of healing can be life-changing, not just for us but also for those around us. As we work on getting better, a strong chance comes up: the opportunity to give back and pay it forward, creating a healing cycle that gives others strength. You don't have to do anything big to show care; small acts of kindness can make a big difference in someone's life.

Sharing What You Know

Think about Michael, who got better from a crippling long-term illness by changing what he ate. Because he has seen how food has changed his own health, Michael wants to share what he knows with other people. He starts a blog where he writes about his journey, gives advice on how to find food triggers, and looks for anti-inflammatory recipes. By talking about his thoughts and experiences, Michael offers hope to people who are going through similar things.

You can share what you know in these ways.

Share your experiences, thoughts, and resources to reach more people. Give advice and connect with people who are going through similar things. Tell people your story and offer support.

What Empathy Can Do for You

Sharing our stories not only helps others learn but also makes us more empathetic and understanding. When we talk about our problems, we make room for others to do the same, which builds community and a shared sense of openness. Feeling like you fit can be very empowering for people who are on their way to healing.

Kind Deeds, No Matter How Small

It's not necessary to make big moves to pay it forward. Being there for someone and listening without judging them can be the most helpful thing you can do. Helping out by running errands, making a healthy meal, or just lending a hand can relieve stress and show your support. Find someone new who is going through the same healing process as you and use your own experiences to help and support them.

Building a Community That Helps Each Other

By paying it forward, we help make the world a better place by being more kind and helpful. Make people more aware of certain health problems and work for better access to help and treatment options. Make it possible for people on similar healing paths to meet each other and make friends. Give your time or skills to groups that help people with health problems.

The Effects of Healing That Spread

Every act of kindness, every bit of information shared, and every moment of help sends out waves. It gives other people the tools they need to heal, builds community, and leads to a world where healing is easier and more caring. Remember that you can make a change even if you don't know everything. Sharing your journey while being open and ready to help can lead to a chain reaction of support and health.

Keep in mind that giving back and paying it forward can change your life as you continue your own mending journey. Please help others by sharing your experiences and encouraging them. This will help build a community where healing can grow.

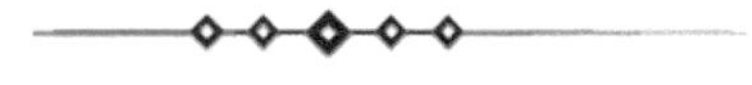

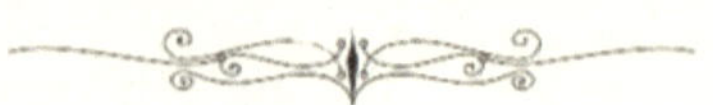

CHAPTER 15

Nourishing Delight

"Recipes for Recovery"

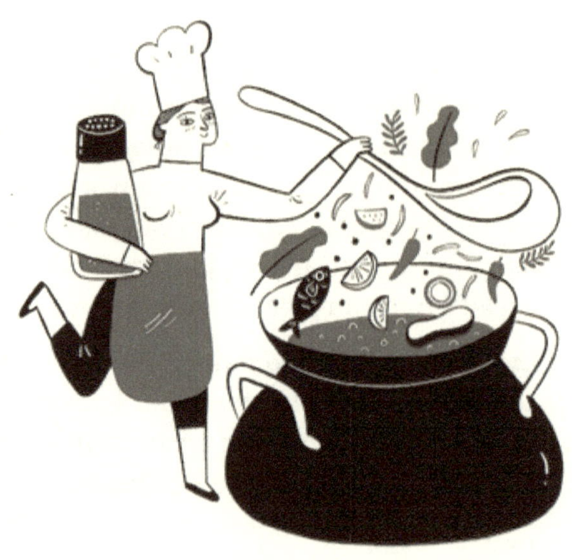

Delicious Doesn't Have to Be Difficult

"Explore a Collection of Easy-to-Follow, Delicious Recipes Specifically Designed to Support Healing"

On the path to healing, nourishing your body with delicious, wholesome food becomes an act of self-love and a powerful tool for recovery. But navigating dietary restrictions or simply finding the time to cook healthy meals can feel like a daunting task. Fear not! This collection of easy-to-follow, flavor-packed recipes is designed to support your healing journey without sacrificing taste or convenience.

Kickstart Your Day with Vibrant Smoothies:

Blend frozen berries, spinach, banana, and almond milk for a refreshing start. This smoothie is packed with vitamins and minerals that support overall well-being. Combine cucumber, green apple, avocado, and kefir (a fermented milk drink rich in gut-friendly probiotics) for a delicious and gut-friendly option.

Nourishing Salads for a Light and Flavorful Lunch

This protein-packed salad features quinoa, chickpeas, roasted vegetables, and a tangy lemon vinaigrette. It's a satisfying and balanced meal perfect for busy weekdays.

A colorful salad packed with anti-inflammatory ingredients like leafy greens, roasted beets, walnuts, and a creamy avocado dressing supports a healthy inflammatory response.

Easy Weeknight Dinners Packed with Flavor

This simple sheet pan dinner features flaky salmon seasoned with lemon and garlic alongside colorful roasted vegetables like broccoli and asparagus. It's a fuss-free and healthy meal ready in under 30 minutes. This hearty and flavorful soup is packed with protein from white beans and fiber from kale. It's a comforting and nourishing option for chilly evenings.

Comfort Food Reimagined: Delicious and Healing

A classic stir-fry gets a healthy makeover with lean chicken, colorful vegetables, and brown rice. It's a satisfying and customizable meal that allows you to incorporate your favorite healing ingredients. This light and flavorful dish features spiralized zucchini noodles tossed in a creamy garlic sauce with fresh spring vegetables. It's a delicious and healthy alternative to traditional pasta dishes.

Don't Forget Dessert! Sweet Treats to Satisfy Your Cravings

This warm and comforting dessert features baked apples stuffed with a mixture of cinnamon, chopped walnuts, and a touch of honey. It's a naturally sweet and satisfying way to end a meal. For a healthy and satisfying snack or dessert, try chia seed pudding. Chia seeds are rich in fiber and omega-3 fatty acids and this pudding is easily customizable with your favorite fruits and nuts.

Beyond the Recipes: Tips for Easy and Healthy Cooking

Dedicate some time on the weekend to chop vegetables, cook grains, and portion out ingredients for the week. This makes grabbing healthy meals throughout the week a breeze. Cook double or triple batches of certain dishes like soups or stews. This allows for leftovers throughout the week and saves you time in the kitchen. Stock your pantry with healthy staples like canned beans, whole grains, and frozen vegetables. These ingredients can be easily transformed into quick and nutritious meals. Frozen fruits and vegetables are flash-frozen at peak ripeness, preserving their nutrients. They're a convenient and affordable way to incorporate fruits and vegetables into your diet. Instead of white rice, opt for brown rice or quinoa. Replace sugary drinks with water or herbal tea. These small changes can significantly boost the nutritional value of your meals.

Food as a Celebration

Eating healthy doesn't have to be a solitary pursuit. Sharing delicious and nourishing meals with loved ones can be a source of joy and connection. Explore different cuisines or dietary styles to create exciting menus. Let family or friends help with meal prep or setting the table. This fosters a sense of shared responsibility and creates a fun experience. Take the time to plate your food thoughtfully and create a welcoming atmosphere at the table. Put away phones and create a space for meaningful conversation. Sharing stories and laughter over a delicious meal strengthens bonds and creates lasting memories. Organize a potluck with friends or family, encouraging everyone to bring a healthy dish. This allows for variety and reduces the burden on one person. Birthdays, holidays, or anniversaries can still be celebrated with delicious food. Options for healthier versions of traditional dishes or introduce new, exciting options. Cooking and sharing meals with loved ones are an opportunity to connect, create traditions, and celebrate the joy of nourishing your body and soul. These shared experiences can be a powerful motivator on your healing journey, fostering a sense of community and support.

The Final Bite: Embrace the Journey of Nourishing Yourself

Healing is a journey, not a destination. There will be days when elaborate meals seem daunting. Embrace these moments and focus on simple, nourishing options. The key is to find a sustainable approach to healthy eating that fits your lifestyle and preferences.

This collection of recipes offers a starting point, but don't be afraid to experiment and personalize them. Explore new ingredients, discover healthy cooking techniques, and, most importantly, have fun in the kitchen! By embracing the joy of cooking and celebrating the power of food to nourish your body and connect with loved ones, you'll be well on your way to a healthier and happier you.

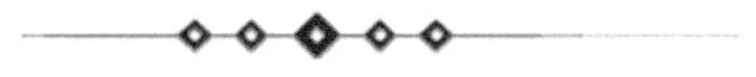

CHAPTER 16

Social Butterfly on a Healing Journey

"Navigating the Social Landscape"

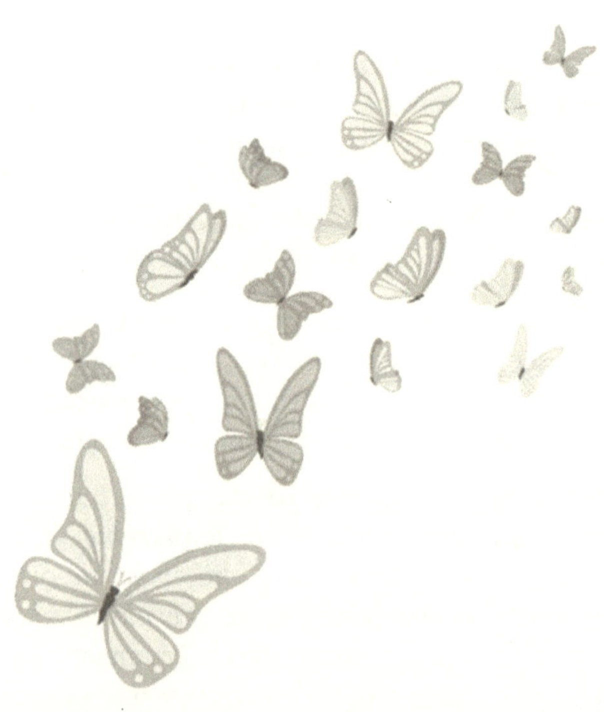

Dining Out Without Derailment

"How to Stay on Track in Social Situations and Restaurants"

Social events and meal trips are important ways for people to connect with each other. But for people who want to stay healthy and heal, it can be hard to handle these situations while keeping their food in mind. Do not be afraid! Here are some ways to handle social settings and restaurants while still following your diet:

Getting ready is key

Look up meals ahead of time. A lot of places put their menus and nutrition facts online. This lets you choose healthy choices ahead of time that fit with your goals. If you're not sure about portion sizes or whether healthy options will be available, bring a small, healthy snack like fruit or nuts to keep yourself from giving in to unhealthy cravings. Water before, during, and after a meal can help you feel full and keep you from eating too much.

Ordering with Mind

Whole, raw foods are better for you than refined carbs and sugary drinks. Lean protein, veggies, and whole grains are what you should eat. Most places are happy to change dishes to fit people with special dietary needs. Find out about the products, how to cook them, and what you can use instead. By ordering smaller amounts or appetizers, you can avoid eating too much. If you're still hungry, you can always ask for more. Putting up healthy walls against people who try to sell you food and social pressure

At social events

People may give you tips you didn't ask for and put pressure on you to indulge. Politely talk about your food tastes and goals. Saying something like "I'm trying to eat healthy right now" or "Thanks" is enough. Suggest hobbies or choices that are better for you. You could suggest going for a walk after dinner or talking over food. Change the subject or focus on the good things about the get-together, like sharing time with family and friends. A funny comment like "My willpower is on a strict diet!" can take the edge off of things and make things easier.

Finding Your Tribe: Making Friends with People Who Share Your Values

It can make a huge difference to be around people who understand and support your journey. Look into online boards or social media groups that are all about healthy eating or certain dietary needs. This lets you connect with other people who are going through the same things. Look for support groups in your area that focus on healthy eating or your health issue. These groups give people a safe place to talk about their problems, get support, and make real relationships. Find family or friends who care about good eating as much as you do. Plan trips or events that focus on cooking classes or learning about healthy foods.

The Power of Having Similar Values

Having family and friends who understand and back your healthy eating choices makes you more responsible and enjoy the process more. Doing social things that involve healthy eating, like cooking lessons or potlucks with nutritious food, can help you stick to your plan and make memories that will last a lifetime. Going out to eat once in a while won't stop you from making progress. Try to make healthy choices as much as possible, but enjoy the odd treat. Pay attention to when you feel hungry or full. Do not feel like you have to finish everything that you have to do. Think about how good you feel and the good changes you're making.

You can feel comfortable in restaurants and social situations if you plan ahead, set healthy limits, and find people who can help you. If you want to stick to your health goals, remember that food can bring you joy and bring people together. Enjoy this trip and all the tasty and healthy things that are waiting for you.

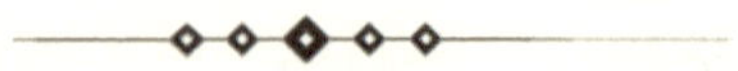

CHAPTER 17

The Magic of Synergy

"Unveiling the Alchemy of Food Combinations"

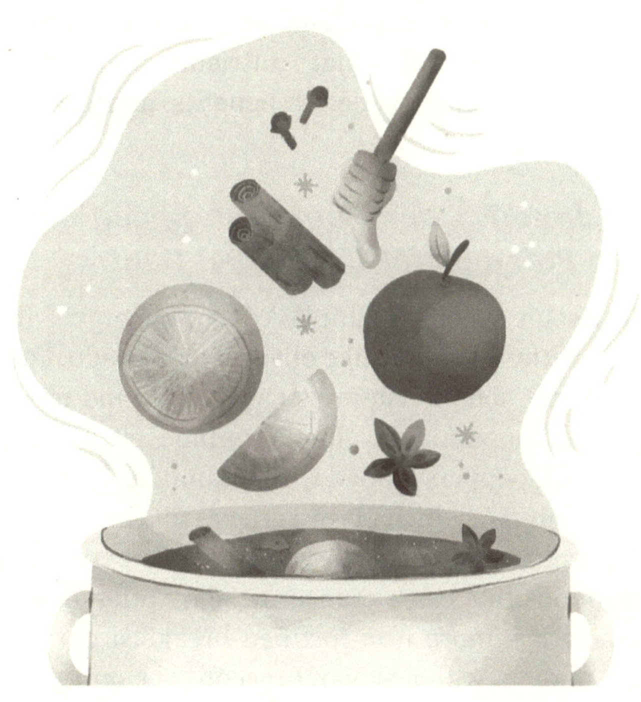

The Power of Food Pairing

"Unlocking Hidden Potential Through Synergy"

Food is more than just sustenance; it's a symphony of flavors and nutrients. But did you know that combining certain foods can unlock a hidden potential, enhancing their nutritional benefits and creating a more powerful impact on your health? This concept is known as food synergy, and it's a fascinating area of food science waiting to be explored.

Understanding Food Synergy

Imagine a team of superheroes. Each hero has unique strengths, but when they join forces, their combined power becomes something truly formidable. Food synergy works similarly. When certain foods are paired together, their individual nutrients interact, enhancing absorption, promoting specific health benefits, and maximizing their overall impact.

Unlocking Hidden Potential: Specific Food Pairings for Enhanced Health

Let's delve into some specific examples of food synergy. Pair your leafy greens with a healthy fat source like olive oil or avocado. Fat helps your body absorb the fat-soluble vitamins (A, K, E) found in leafy greens, maximizing their nutritional value. Combine citrus fruits rich in vitamin C with bell peppers loaded with vitamin A. Vitamin C aids the absorption of vitamin A, which plays a crucial role in immune function. Enjoy your morning oatmeal with a sprinkle of berries. The berries contain compounds that can enhance the absorption of iron from the oatmeal, making it a more iron-fortified breakfast option. Pair your fatty fish, like salmon, with a side of broccoli. The omega-3 fatty acids in the fish can help protect the delicate vitamin C found in broccoli, creating a potent antioxidant duo.

Creating Flavorful and Synergistic Meals: Putting It All Together

Now that you understand the concept of food synergy let's get creative! Don't just throw lettuce and tomatoes on a plate. Add a dollop of olive oil, sprinkle some chopped walnuts, and top it with berries for a symphony of textures and a boost of healthy fats, vitamin E, and antioxidants. Combine lean chicken or tofu with colorful vegetables like broccoli and peppers. Throw in some cashew nuts for added protein and healthy fats, creating a complete and nutrient-rich meal. Don't underestimate the power of a well-crafted soup. Pure roasted butternut squash with carrots and ginger. A dollop of coconut milk adds a touch of creaminess and healthy fats, while the ginger helps with nutrient absorption.

These are just a few examples. Experiment with different flavor combinations and explore the world of food synergy. With a little creativity, you can turn your meals into delicious and powerful tools for optimal health.

The Final Bite: Food Pairing: A Journey of Exploration

Food pairing is an exciting journey of discovery. As you explore different combinations, you'll not only unlock the hidden potential of your food but also create a more dynamic and enjoyable culinary experience. So, embrace the power of food synergy, experiment with flavors, and let your kitchen become a haven for delicious and health-promoting meals!

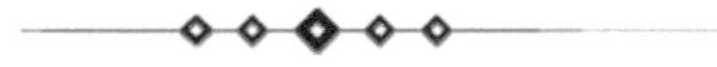

CHAPTER 18

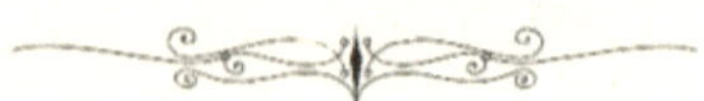

A Glimpse into the Future

"The Future of Nutrition in Recovery"

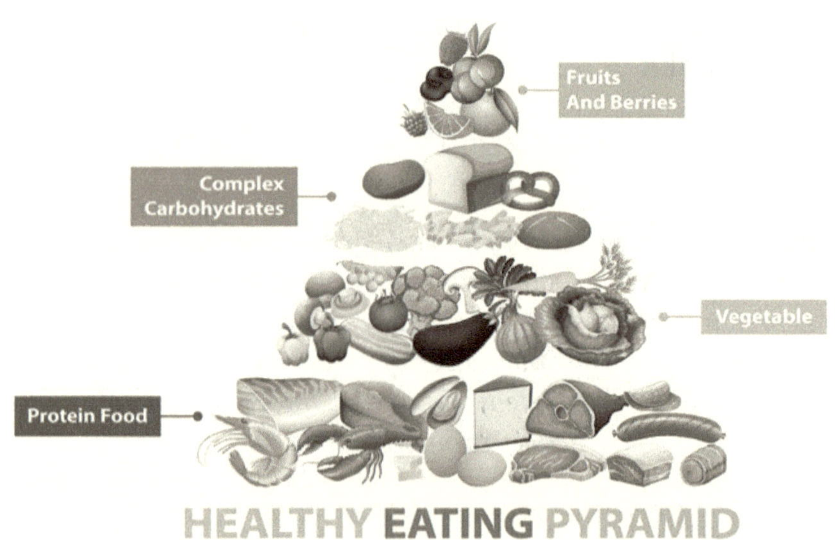

New Technologies and Trends

A Look at the Future of Food and Health"

The field of nutrition is always changing, and exciting new discoveries are changing how we think about food and health. As you work on your healing, knowing about these new tools and trends can help you take a more proactive and personalized approach to your health. Personalized nutrition is becoming more popular, and it can help you stay healthy. Gone are the days when there was one diet that worked for everyone. Personalized nutrition uses cutting-edge tools like genetic tests, gut microbiome analysis, and wearable health trackers to make diet plans that are specific to your needs and biometrics.

What Could Happen to Recovery

Personalized nutrition can help you figure out what nutrients you might be missing or sensitive to so you can focus on eating certain foods or taking certain pills to help your body heal. Gut health is very important for general health. Personalized suggestions based on an analysis of your gut microbiome can help improve your digestion, absorption of nutrients, and general recovery. Wearable health trackers show you your blood sugar levels, sleep habits, and activity levels in real time. When combined with personalized meal plans, this information lets changes and improvements be made for better recovery results.

The Rise of Functional Foods: Food as Medicine

Functional foods are a trend in the food business that is growing very quickly. These foods are more than just good for you; they also have extra health benefits that help with certain body processes or keep you from getting sick. These good bacteria help keep your gut healthy and your immune system strong. Some foods that are naturally high in probiotics are yogurt, kimchi, and kombucha. Prebiotics feed the good bacteria in your gut, which helps them grow and do their job. Prebiotics can be found in lots of foods, such as onions, garlic, and chicory root. This group of mushrooms and herbs helps the body deal with stress and feel better all around. Ashwagandha, Rhodiola rosea, and reishi mushrooms are some examples.

What Could Happen to Recovery

You can add functional foods to your diet to help with certain things you need as you heal. As an example, probiotics can help keep your gut healthy after taking antibiotics, and adaptogens can help you deal with stress and sleep better. Eating different useful foods together can make them work better together, making them healthier overall. It's getting easier to add functional foods to your diet because they are becoming more common in grocery stores and online.

Food as Medicine for Prevention: Going Beyond Recovery

Functional foods and a personalized diet are very important for healing, but they can be used for many other things as well. Personalized eating plans can help you avoid future health problems and stay healthy in the long term by taking into account your specific needs and risk factors. Wearable health trackers and blood sugar tracking systems can show early signs of possible health problems so they can be stopped or treated quickly. Personalized nutrition systems can look at your genes and other biometrics to figure out how likely it is that you will get certain health problems. This knowledge lets people make changes to their diet and way of life that can help prevent disease.

Challenges and Things to Think About

These advances open up a lot of exciting options, such as personalized nutrition services, genetic tests, and some functional foods, which can be pricey, and not everyone may be able to get their hands on them easily. The market for functional foods is still growing, so rules about claims and quality control are needed to protect consumers and make sure the products work. Personalization tools for nutrition gather a lot of information about your health. It is very important to understand data privacy standards and make sure your information is safe.

What's Next for Food and Healing?

Personalized, useful, and preventative food is the way of the future. Innovative food products and new technologies have a huge amount of promise to speed up the healing process and improve overall health. Staying informed about these changes and smartly accepting them can give you the power to take charge of your health and build a healthy, strong future.

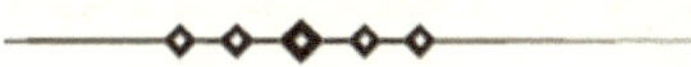

CHAPTER 19

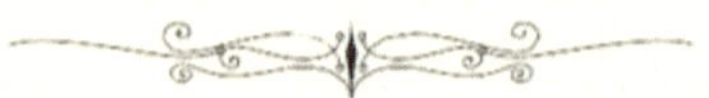

Beyond Food

"Integrating Lifestyle Changes for Comprehensive Healing"

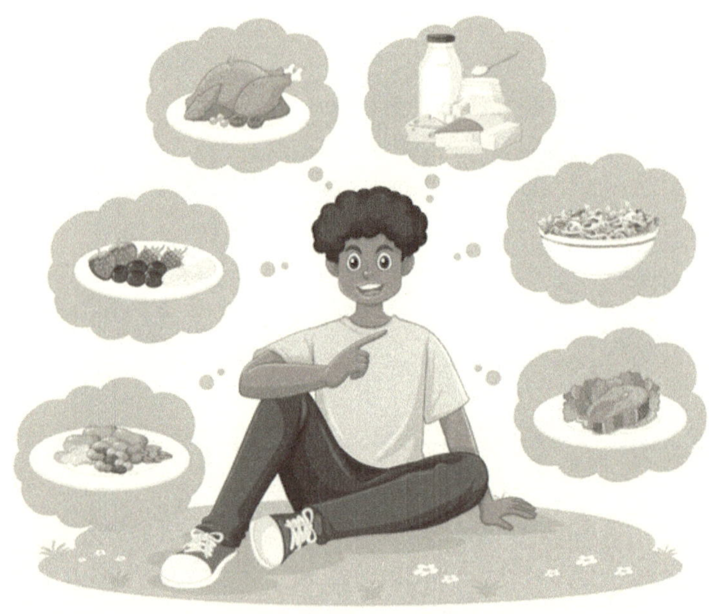

Sleep is the basis of healing.

"How to use the healing power of restorative sleep."

Prioritize one thing above all else while you're healing: good sleep. It's not a luxury to get enough sleep; it's a basic need for good health and healing. While you sleep, your body heals tissues, gets energy back, and makes memories stronger. Why sleep is important and how to get a good night's rest:

Why Good Sleep Is Important

Your body does a lot of different repair work while you sleep. You can heal fast- er because your muscles and organs repair themselves, and your immune system gets stronger. Lack of sleep can make it harder to concentrate, remember things, and control your emotions. Getting enough sleep helps you think more clearly, feel better, and deal with worry better. Your body controls chemicals like growth hormones while you sleep. Growth hormone is very important for cell growth and repair. Getting enough sleep also helps keep cortisol levels in a healthy range. Cortisol is a stress hormone that, if too high, can slow down healing.

What You Can Do to Get Restorative Sleep

Set a regular sleep schedule. Even on the weekends, I go to bed and wake up at the same time every day. This helps keep your body's normal sleep-wake cycle in balance, which makes it easier to fall asleep and feel better when you wake up. Do things that calm you down before bed, like taking a warm bath, reading a book, or doing some light yoga poses. Electronic devices give off blue light that can make it hard to sleep, so don't use screens for at least an hour before bed. Make sure your bedroom is dark, quiet, and cool to get the best sleep possible. Buy soft bedding and a cushion that will support your body. Don't drink or use coffee in the evening because it can make it hard to fall asleep. Regular exercise can help you sleep better for longer. But don't do any hard workouts right before bed. Meditation and deep breathing exercises are two mindfulness practices that can help you calm down and get ready for sleep.

Managing stress is the missing piece in getting better.

Stress can be good and bad at the same time. Hormones that slow down heal-ing can be released by worry, and long-term stress can make health problems worse. Learning how to deal with stress is an important part of getting better. To calm your nervous system and deal with stress, try deep breathing techniques, progressive muscle relaxation, or meditation. Mindfulness practices, such as writing in a book or spending time in nature, can help you become more aware of your feelings and thoughts, which can help you better handle them. The type of treatment called cognitive behavioral therapy (CBT) can help you figure out and change the negative thought patterns that make you feel stressed. Surround yourself with positive, helpful people who understand the problems you're facing and can offer support.

Movement is Life: Finding Gentle Exercises to Help You Heal

During some stages of healing, it may not be a good idea to do intense exercises, but gentle moving routines can be very helpful. Regular exercise, like light yoga or walks, makes the blood flow better. This gives your cells the nutrients and oxygen they need to repair and heal. Light exercise can help people with certain illnesses deal with pain. Endorphins are natural chemicals that make you feel better and can help your general health. Being active is a natural way to release stress. Light exercise can help control stress hormones and make you feel cool and relaxed. Working out regularly can help keep your sleep cycle in check, which can make it easier to fall asleep and stay asleep all night.

By getting enough good sleep, dealing with stress well, and doing some light exercise every day, you'll build a strong base for healing. Don't forget that healing is a process, not a goal. Be kind to yourself, enjoy the little wins, and know that sleep, managing stress, and exercise can help you feel better.

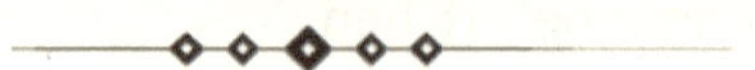

CHAPTER 20

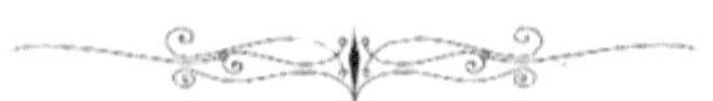

Building Your Blueprint for Recovery

"Navigating Wellness"

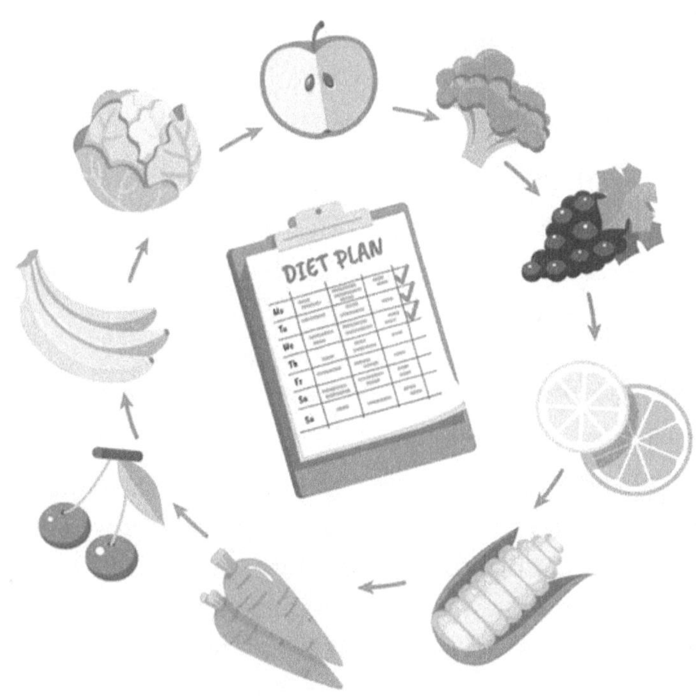

Goal Setting for Success

"Charting Your Course on the Healing Journey"

Navigating a healing journey requires both determination and a roadmap for success. That's where effective goal setting comes in. Setting clear, achievable goals will keep you motivated, focused, and empowered to celebrate your progress.

The Power of SMART Goals

Specific: Instead of a vague goal like "get healthier," define a particular objective, such as "walk for 30 minutes, 3 times a week."

Measurable: How will you track your progress? Are you aiming for a specific number of steps, a certain amount of weight loss, or improved sleep quality?

Attainable: Set challenging yet achievable goals. Unrealistic goals can lead to discouragement. Start small and gradually increase the difficulty as you progress.

Relevant: Align your goals with your overall health goals and recovery needs.

Time-bound: Set a timeline for achieving your goals. This creates a sense of urgency and helps you track your progress.

Beyond SMART Goals: Creating a Personalized Plan

What aspects of your health do you want to focus on? Nutrition, sleep, stress management, or physical activity? Break down your long-term vision into smaller, manageable short-term goals. Celebrate achieving these milestones, and use them as stepping stones towards your larger goals. There will be setbacks and days when motivation wanes. Forgive yourself, learn from setbacks, and recommit to your goals. The key is to focus on overall progress, not occasional slip-ups.

Creating a Sustainable Plan: Building Lifelong Habits

Your healing journey is a marathon, not a sprint. Find ways to make healthy habits enjoyable. Cooking with friends, exploring new hiking trails, or joining a fitness class with a positive environment. Surround yourself with positive and supportive people who encourage your health goals. Life throws curveballs. Adapt your plan as needed, but don't give up on your overall goals.

Celebrating Every Milestone: The Power of Self-Compassion

During your healing journey, celebrating your achievements, big or small, is crucial. Recognizing progress reinforces positive behaviors and motivates you to keep going. Celebrating your victories builds self-confidence and strengthens your ability to achieve your goals. Taking the time to acknowledge your efforts helps reduce stress, making the journey more manageable.

Embrace Self-Compassion

Be kind to yourself. Healing is a journey, not a destination. There will be days when you stumble. Forgive yourself, learn from setbacks, and use them as opportunities to grow. Focus on the positive changes you're making, celebrate your victories, and maintain a positive outlook.

Goal setting is a journey, not a destination. Revisit and adapt your goals as needed. Celebrate every milestone, big or small. Your progress deserves recognition. Practice self-compassion throughout the healing journey. Be kind to yourself and acknowledge your efforts. By creating a personalized plan and celebrating your progress, you'll be well on your way to a successful and sustainable healing journey. Embrace the challenges, celebrate your victories, and remember – you've got this!

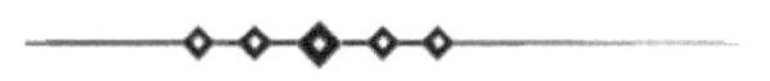

Closing Thoughts

I hope that this book has helped you on your way to healing. Remember that healing doesn't happen in a straight line. There will be good days and bad days, times when you feel eager and times when you're not. You can get through these problems and come out better and healthier if you have the right tools and help. These recipes are just a place to begin; they're meant to inspire you to be creative and try new things. As you play around with different flavors and ingredients, don't forget to focus on whole, healthy foods that help your body heal itself. It would help if you weren't afraid to switch things out or make changes based on your food wants and preferences. Don't forget that food is more than just fuel; it's also a way to meet, have fun, and celebrate. Sharing healthy, tasty meals with people you care about can be a powerful way to boost your mood and keep you going. Explore the world of food unity outside of the kitchen to find out how to combine foods in ways that make them healthier. Take advantage of the great new developments in personalized nutrition and useful foods, and learn how they can help you take charge of your health. Lastly, make sure you get enough good sleep, learn how to deal with stress well, and include gentle movement in your daily life.

With these basic techniques, you can build a strong base for healing and well-being. Being kind to yourself is the most important thing during this process. Honor every achievement, no matter how big or small. Forgive yourself when things go wrong, and use them to learn. It takes time, work, and kindness to yourself to heal. This e-book is the first step. You can be as healthy and happy as possible if you commit to good habits, keep a positive attitude, and get help from people you care about. Believe that you can get better—you have the power to make your future bright and healthy.

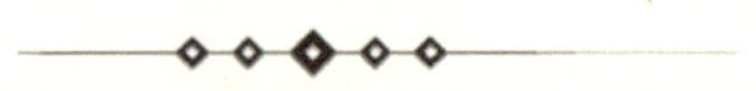